CULTURAL ISSUES IN THE TREATMENT OF ANXIETY

Cultural Issues in the Treatment of Anxiety

Edited by

STEVEN FRIEDMAN

THE GUILFORD PRESS
New York London

©1997 The Guilford Press
A Division of Guilford Publications, Inc.
72 Spring Street, New York, NY 10012

Printed in the United States of America

This book is printed on acid-free paper.

Last digit is print number: 9 8 7 6 5 4 3 2 1

Library of Congress Cataloging-in-Publication Data

Cultural issues in the treatment of anxiety / edited by Steven
 Friedman.
     p.   cm.
 Based on a one day symposium. "Recognizing and treating
anxiety disorders across cultures": sponsored by the Dept. of
Psychiatry, State University of New York Health Science Center
at Brooklyn, Dec. 1995.
   Includes bibliographical references and index.
   ISBN 1-57230-237-2
   1. Anxiety—Cross-cultural studies. 2. Psychiatry,
Transcultural. I. Friedman, Steven, 1954.
   RC531.C85 1997
   616.85′223—dc21   97–13509
                                                              CIP

Contributors

Robert Ackerman, MSW, Clinical Instructor, Department of Psychiatry, State University of New York Health Science Center at Brooklyn, Brooklyn, NY

Anwarul Ahad, MD, Clinical Instructor, Department of Psychiatry, State University of New York Health Science Center at Brooklyn, Brooklyn, NY

Janet Brice-Baker, PhD, Assistant Professor, Department of Psychology, Yeshiva University, Bronx, NY

Kimberly Diamond, BS, Research Assistant, New York State Psychiatric Institute, Columbia University, New York, NY

Steven Friedman, PhD, Professor of Clinical Psychiatry, Department of Psychiatry, State University of New York Health Science Center at Brooklyn, Brooklyn, NY

Jack M. Gorman, MD, Professor of Clinical Psychiatry, Department of Psychiatry, Columbia University College of Physicans and Surgeons, New York, NY

Peter J. Guarnaccia, PhD, Associate Professor, Institute for Health, Health Care Policy, and Aging Research, Rutgers University, New Brunswick, NJ

Marjorie L. Hatch, PhD, Assistant Professor, Department of Psychology, Southern Methodist University, Dallas, TX

Ewald Horwath, MD, Associate Clinical Professor of Psychiatry, Department of Psychiatry, Columbia University College of Physicians and Surgeons, New York, NY

94834

Gayle Y. Iwamasa, PhD, Assistant Professor, Department of Psychology, Oklahoma State University, Stillwater, OK

Carlos Jusino, MD, Research Psychiatrist, New York State Psychiatric Institute, Columbia University, New York, NY

Laurence J. Kirmayer, MD, Professor and Director, Division of Social and Transcultural Psychiatry, McGill University, Montreal, Quebec, and Institute of Community and Family Psychiatry, Sir Mortimer B. Davis–Jewish General Hospital, Montreal, Quebec

Arturo Sánchez-LaCay, MD, Research Psychiatrist, New York State Psychiatric Institute, Columbia University, New York, NY

Ira M. Lesser, MD, Professor, Department of Psychiatry, Harbor–UCLA Research Center on the Psychobiology of Ethnicity, Torrance, CA

Michael R. Liebowitz, MD, Professor of Clinical Psychiatry and Director, Anxiety Disorders Clinic, New York State Psychiatric Institute, Columbia University, New York, NY

Keh-Ming Lin, MPH, MD, Professor, Department of Psychiatry and Biobehavioral Sciences, UCLA School of Medicine, and Director, Harbor–UCLA Research Center on the Psychobiology of Ethnicity, Torrance, CA

Sharon-ann Gopaul McNicol, PhD, Professor, School of Education, Howard University, Washington, DC

Angela M. Neal-Barnett, PhD, Associate Professor, Department of Psychology, Kent State University, Kent, OH

Cheryl M. Paradis, PsyD, Clinical Associate Professor, Department of Psychiatry, State University of New York Health Science Center at Brooklyn, Brooklyn, NY

Russell E. Poland, PhD, Department of Psychiatry, Harbor–UCLA Research Center on the Psychobiology of Ethnicity, Torrance, CA

Ester Salmán, BS, Research Administrator, Hispanic Treatment Program, Anxiety Disorders Clinic, New York State Psychiatric Institute, Columbia University, New York, NY

Jeffrey Smith, Sr., MA, MEd, Department of Psychology, Kent State University Kent, OH

Manoj R. Shah, MD, Assistant Professor of Psychiatry, Albert Einstein College of Medicine, Bronx, NY, and Department of Psychiatry, Long Island Jewish–Hillside Medical Center, Queens, NY

Michael Smith, MD, Department of Psychiatry, Harbor–UCLA Research Center on the Psychobiology of Ethnicity, Torrance, CA

Ramaswamy Viswanathan, MD, DSc, Associate Professor of Clinical Psychiatry, Department of Psychiatry, State University of New York Health Science Center at Brooklyn, Brooklyn, NY

Myrna M. Weissman, PhD, Professor of Epidemiology in Psychiatry, Columbia University College of Physicians and Surgeons and Chief, Division of Clinical and Genetic Epidemiology, New York State Psychiatric Institute, Columbia University, New York, NY

Lawrence A. Welkowitz, PhD, Research Scientist, New York State Psychiatric Institute, Columbia University, New York, NY, and Assistant Professor, Department of Psychology, Keene State College, Keene, NH

Acknowledgments

This book emanates in part from a 1-day symposium on treating anxiety disorders across cultures that was held at the State University of New York Health Science Center at Brooklyn on December 7, 1995. This volume would not be possible without the active support and encouragement of numerous individuals. The conference itself was supported in part by unrestricted educational grants from Wyeth–Ayerst, Janssen, and Upjohn.

Russell L. Miller, MD, President of the State University of New York Health Science Center at Brooklyn, and Ross Clinchy, PhD, Assistant to the President, ensured that the administration of the university, through the Arthur Ashe Institute for Urban Health (Ruth C. Browne, Director), lent much needed assistance. Eugene B. Feigelson, MD, Chairman of the Department of Psychiatry and Dean of the College of Medicine, has historically been the driving force in establishing the Anxiety Disorders Clinic at our university. Over the years, he has been instrumental in ensuring that all patients, regardless of ability to pay, obtained appropriate, state-of-the-art treatment. His continued support of our clinic and this conference is greatly appreciated. Numerous faculty members of the Department of Psychiatry offered their advice and feedback. In particular, Cheryl M. Paradis, PsyD, was extremely helpful in all aspects of planning the conference as well as this volume. She was especially gracious in reading all submissions to this volume and offering her feedback.

Members of the Anxiety Disorders Clinic staff, Robert Ackerman, MSW, Marjorie Hatch, PhD, Cheryl M. Paradis, PsyD, Lisa Smith, MA, Brian Trappler, MD, and Ramaswamy Viswanathan, MD, have long been sources of collegial support. I would especially like to thank Barbara Singh, who has been my right hand in providing secretarial and administrative support in planning the conference and preparing this volume. Catherine Cozzolino has also consistently lent a hand in this effort. I also would like to thank Seymour Weingarten, Editor-in-Chief, and Jeannie Tang, Production Editor, at The Guilford Press.

I have learned much from the many teachers and supervisors who have guided my training and thinking. Looking back, I owe a personal debt of gratitude to the State University of New York at Stony Brook, where I obtained my training in clinical psychology. The faculty's commitment to empirical and clinical research has greatly influenced my own approach to clinical problems. In particular, I would like to thank Gerald C. Davidson and Marvin Goldfried, who, as my graduate advisors, served as role models in sharpening my skills in the observation of human behavior and in encouraging the development of the best possible treatment for our clients.

On a personal note, I would like to thank my wife, Miriam, and children, Bonnie, Stuart, Abraham, and Raphael, for their long-term support. Finally, I need to express my deep gratitude to all my patients over the years who have entrusted me with their care. I am continuously amazed at how the process of being involved in providing help for others has enabled me to grow; it has always been a gratifying and rewarding experience as well. I hope this volume will increase knowledge of the anxiety disorders and ensure that the best quality of care is available to all who need it.

Preface

Since the *Diagnostic and Statistical Manual of Mental Disoders,* 3rd edition (DSM-III; American Psychiatric Association, 1980) operationalized the definition of the anxiety disorders and made the critical distinction between panic and other anxiety disorders, the number of studies in this area has dramatically increased. Studies have looked at epidemiological, phenomenological, and genetic factors, as well as patients' responses to behavioral and psychopharmacological treatments. The recent wealth of clinical studies led the National Institutes of Health (1991) to publish guidelines for the treatment of panic disorder.

During the past decade, demographic projections have forecast major changes in the makeup of American society. By the year 2050, forecasters have suggested that more than one half of the population in the United States will be of Hispanic, African American, Asian, or Native American descent. However, as reviewed by Neal and Turner (1991) and others (Friedman, 1994), in the United States, published clinical research data on the diagnosis and treatment of anxiety disorders in cultural groups other than white, middle-class Americans have been rare.

This volume emanates in part from a 1-day symposium, "Recognizing and Treating Anxiety Disorders across Cultures," sponsored by the Department of Psychiatry, State University of New York Health Science Center at Brooklyn, held in December 1995. The focus of that conference was to provide a state-of-the-art review of the evidence available on the diagnosis and treatment of anxiety disorders across different ethnic groups.

Peter J. Guarnaccia begins this volume by providing a cross-cultural perspective on anxiety disorders. As a medical anthropologist with a keen interest in studying anxiety disorders, he provides an overview of the issues one needs to consider when examining anxiety in different ethnic or cultural groups, both within the United States and across the globe. He addresses several key issues, such as the following: What is the frequency of anxiety disorders worldwide? Are there different risk factors for anxiety across ethnic groups? Are there differences in symptom patterns across cultures? Are there culture-specific syndromes or idioms of distress that might fit DSM-IV (fourth edition) anxiety disorders? Is posttraumatic stress disorder an appropriate diagnosis, or does it require modification for refugees from Southeast Asia and Central America? Finally, would the incorporation of a mixed anxiety–depression diagnosis in DSM-IV help in studying and treating cross-cultural expressions of anxiety?

Ewald Horwath and Myrna M. Weissman provide an analysis of the epidemiology of anxiety disorders across cultural groups on the basis of DSM-III or DSM-III-R (3rd edition, revised) criteria. They review the available evidence for the epidemiology of panic disorder, agoraphobia, social phobia, generalized anxiety disorder, and obsessive–compulsive disorder in the United States and worldwide. They also review data on the risk factors for anxiety disorders, such as gender, age, race/ethnicity, and marital and economic status. In addition to showing how prevalent these disorders are, they document how our epidemiological understanding of these disorders has grown over the past several years.

Lawrence A. Welkowitz and Jack M. Gorman complete Part I of this volume by providing a brief overview of the treatment of anxiety disorders, focusing on the treatment of panic disorder as a model. Cognitive-behavioral and psychopharmacological approaches have been empirically shown to be quite effective in the treatment of panic disorder, and the authors review issues in the pathophysiology, assessment, and treatment of this disorder.

In Part II of this book, I invited a number of authors to provide an overview of the treatment of anxiety in different ethnic groups. In order to provide some consistency among chapters, the authors were asked to organize their chapters around some common themes. Specific issues included the following: How does this cultural group view "mental illness" and "anxiety"? How does this group view psychological or psychiatric treatment? Are there specific anxiety symptoms unique to this group? What are some key points for the clinician to consider in arriving at an accurate diagnosis and establishing a working alliance? What does the literature say about these issues? Are there specific needs that must be addressed beyond the "usual state-of-the-art treatment"? I believe that all of these authors admirably address these points.

In examining issues in the treatment of Hispanic Americans, Ester Salmán, Kimberly Diamond, Carlos Jusino, Arturo Sánchez-LaCay, and Michael R. Liebowitz draw upon their experience at the Hispanic Treatment Program at the New York State Psychiatric Institute. They review a variety of important issues such as the growing Hispanic population in the United States, the limited number of bilingual–bicultural mental health specialists, and patients' levels of acculturation. The authors also address how these issues impact the patient's view of mental illness and of seeking help for anxiety symptoms. The authors also review the culture-bound syndromes of *ataque de nervios* and *nervios*. They briefly review their experience in using medications with this population and provide an overview on their use of a culturally sensitive interview that they believe helps engage this traditionally treatment-resistant population.

Sharon-ann Gopaul-McNicol and Janet Brice-Baker address the issues in treating Caribbean immigrants, who comprise a particular subgroup of African Americans. They provide an overview of this group's view of mental illness and psychotherapy. The authors discuss possible risk factors for the development of anxiety disorders in this population and, finally, provide the clinician with some principles of assessment and treatment. In particular, they emphasize the need to understand the structure of Caribbean families and how it is often necessary to engage the entire family in the treatment process.

Gayle Y. Iwamasa provides a thorough review of the cultural similarities and differences within the Asian American community. She touches upon a wide range of demographic and clinical variables such as ethnic identity, language, acculturation, immigrant status, religion, gender roles, and cultural traditions. These variables will obviously affect patients' help-seeking behavior and their view of their symptoms. She reviews for the clinician a number of important issues for assessment and treatment with this population, such as the extent of somatization, depression, and alcohol and drug use, as well as the impact of symptoms on interpersonal relationships. Her outline of the issues involved in treating Asian Americans can serve as a checklist for the clinician. Proper attention paid to these variables will increase the probability of engaging and keeping the patient in treatment.

Cheryl M. Paradis, Steven Friedman, Marjorie L. Hatch, and Robert Ackerman review the treatment of Orthodox Jews. As we note, this religious group is a minority even within the overall Jewish community in the United States. However, some of the issues we raise in treating this devoutly religious group may be similar to the treatment of other religious groups such as Muslims, Mormons, and Seventh Day Adventists. Historically, mental health professionals have either neglected or had a negative view of the role of a patient's religious beliefs in the assessment and treatment of emotional problems (Shafranske, 1996). It is hoped that this chapter will serve as a catalyst for examining the role of religion, a neglected area of clinical research, in the diagnosis and treatment of anxiety disorders.

Following the influential review of Neal and Turner (1991) there has been growth, albeit limited, in the literature on African Americans with anxiety disorders, primarily focusing on panic disorder in adults and fears/phobias in children. In their chapter, Angela M. Neal-Barnett and Jeffrey Smith, Sr., review the literature on panic disorder, generalized anxiety disorder, and obsessive–compulsive disorder in the African American community. They note the clinical importance of assessing a variety of areas such as spirituality, the role of extended family, victimization, isolated sleep paralysis, and the therapeutic alliance when engaging African Americans in the treatment of anxiety.

Ramaswamy Viswanathan, Manoj R. Shah, and Anwarul Ahad, in reviewing the issues in treating Asian-Indian Americans, highlight the fact that the world view of people from the Indian subcontinent is more likely to be sociocentric rather than egocentric. Many of the contributors to this volume have described how in the United States, personal autonomy and individuality are highly valued. However, in much of the rest of the world, the group (family, neighbors, and society) is more valued than the individual. The authors of this chapter point out that Indian society, in contrast to that of the United States, is more restrictive and rule bound, with clearly defined gender and hierarchical roles. Privacy is not a priority and behavior is highly influenced by the concept of shame. These values will affect how the initial referral or contact is made. Similarly, patients and their families have clear expectations of the first session and treatment. The clinician needs to be aware of the expectations of the identified patient and his or her family. Viswanathan and colleagues review some culture-specific clinical syndromes and situations, as well as providing some idea of indigenous therapeutic practices and how these will impact the delivery of mental health treatment.

In Part III of this volume, Ira M. Lesser, Michael Smith, Russell E. Poland, and Keh-Ming Lin provide a fascinating overview of the emerging clinical research on psychopharmacological treatment and ethnicity. In their chapter, they begin by outlining some mechanisms governing drug responses and, using this as a background, they go on to cover purported influences of ethnicity and culture on response to psychopharmacological treatment. They review the clinical and research implications of these findings, suggest some clinical guidelines, and provide future research directions. Understanding of the interplay between psychopharmacology and ethnicity is clearly still in the infancy stage and their chapter provides a succinct introduction to and summary of this critically important field.

In the closing chapter of this volume, Laurence J. Kirmayer, in a scholarly and thorough fashion, sets the agenda for clinical and research work on culture and anxiety. He reviews recent work on emotion theory for the place of culture in emotional experience, some evidence for cultural variations in symptoms and mechanisms of anxiety disorders, and some overall clinical issues of relevance to practicing in an increasing ethnically diverse society. His analysis of the concept of posttraumatic stress disorder in DSM-IV forces us to examine the broader social context for anxiety disorders and their treatment.

Clearly, this volume can only briefly highlight some of the important clinical and theoretical issues in such a rich and complex field as the role of culture in anxiety and its treatment. We hope that this volume will make a modest contribution to this important and long-neglected area.

REFERENCES

American Psychiatric Association. (1980). *Diagnostic and statistical-manual of mental disorders* (3rd ed.). Washington, DC: American Psychiatric Association.

Friedman, S. (Ed.). (1994). *Anxiety disorders in African-Americans.* New York: Springer.

Neal, A. M., & Turner, S. M. (1991). Anxiety disorders research with African-Americans: Current status. *Psychological Bulletin, 109,* 400–410.

National Institutes of Health. (1991). Panic consensus statement. *9*(2)

Shafranske, E. P. (Ed.). (1996). *Religion and the clinical practice of psychology.* Washington, DC: American Psychological Association.

Contents

Part III. Special Topics

I

GENERAL ISSUES IN THE CROSS-CULTURAL TREATMENT OF ANXIETY DISORDERS

1

A Cross-Cultural Perspective on Anxiety Disorders

PETER J. GUARNACCIA

STATEMENT AND SIGNIFICANCE OF THE ISSUES

This chapter will examine cultural issues in applying the diagnostic criteria for the anxiety disorders to individuals from different cultural groups both within the United States and across the globe. The major focus of this chapter, then, is on issues of diagnosis of the anxiety disorders across cultures rather than on treatment issues, which will be addressed in later chapters about specific ethnic groups. The chapter builds on three previous reviews of this area: Good and Kleinman's (1985) review of culture and anxiety; my review with Kirmayer (Guarnaccia & Kirmayer, 1997) for Volume 3 of the *DSM-IV Sourcebook*; and a review by Kirmayer and colleagues (1995) in a special issue of *The Psychiatric Clinics of North America* focused on "cultural psychiatry." A key issue in the cross-cultural application of anxiety diagnostic criteria is whether the emotional symptoms of excessive worry or apprehension are necessarily the predominant symptoms and whether they should be given priority over the range of somatic symptoms and rich bodily idioms of anxiety that are often of concern in the cross-cultural literature to people experiencing these disorders.

The importance of examining the interface between culture and anxiety was thoroughly reviewed by Good and Kleinman (1985), who start their review with the following assertion:

> The cross-cultural research . . . makes it abundantly clear that anxiety and disorders of anxiety are universally present in human societies. It makes equally clear that the phenomenology of such disorders, the meaningful forms through which distress is articulated and constituted as social reality, varies in quite significant ways across cultures. (p. 298)

After reviewing the literature available, they conclude that, across cultures, complaints associated with anxiety are articulated through culture-specific idioms. These include a range of "fright" disorders, problems associated with "nerves" and neurasthenia, and a range of somatized expressions of distress. They also note that these "rich somatic idioms have produced difficulties for clinicians and researchers in distinguishing anxiety, depression and somatoform disorders" (p. 311). One of the key goals of this chapter is to provide more detail on assessing anxiety in multicultural patients. This will be an increasingly important issue for clinicians working in the United States as client populations become more culturally diverse and the proportion of recent immigrants increases. Recent projections by the Bureau of the Census suggest that, by the year 2050, 45% of the U.S. population will be composed of persons who are Latinos, African Americans, and Asian Americans.

Good and Kleinman (1985) identify several domains of experience, including fertility, dreams, magical aggression, and witchcraft, that are associated with anxiety and raise "culture-specific questions about the boundaries between normalcy and pathology" (p. 311). Good and Kleinman's review poses a number of questions and issues about the epidemiology, clinical course, and social factors that place people at risk for anxiety disorders. These include the following (Good & Kleinman, 1985, pp. 322–323):

> *The epidemiological question*: What is the frequency and distribution of anxiety disorders worldwide?
>
> *The clinical descriptive question*: What is the relationship of different anxiety disorders to different styles of illness behavior and idioms of distress among distinctive cultures, ethnic groups, and social classes?
>
> *The psychological question*: Are there cross-cultural differences in the cognitive, affective, and communicative processes (such as

attention, perception, affective socialization) that contribute to the development and expression of anxiety disorders?

The social question: What are the social factors that increase risk for anxiety? Are they specific for anxiety or do they hold for mental illness more broadly?

Although the literature since Good and Kleinman's paper addresses many of these issues, a number of their questions remain unresolved.

The purpose of this review will be to update progress on these issues and to specify areas for further research. There has been less attention to the anxiety disorders than to either schizophrenia or depression in cross-cultural research. There has not been a major World Health Organization (WHO) study for anxiety disorders as there has been for schizophrenia (WHO, 1973, 1979) and depression (WHO, 1983), although the current WHO studies of psychopathology in primary care do include the anxiety disorders.

Even in the recent Epidemiologic Catchment Area (ECA) studies (Regier et al., 1984), there has been limited focus on the anxiety disorders in spite of their high prevalence in the population (Karno et al., 1989; Brown, Eaton, & Sussman, 1990). The ECA studies were designed to provide a portrait of the mental health of the American population. Five sites were selected to represent regional, ethnic and residential diversity, including four urban/suburban sites in Baltimore, Maryland, Los Angeles, California, New Haven, Connecticut, and St. Louis, Missouri. The fifth site was more rural in composition and was from the Raleigh–Durham area of North Carolina. Both the Baltimore and St. Louis sites oversampled African Americans and the Los Angeles site oversampled Mexican Americans so that the prevalences of disorder could be estimated for these important multicultural populations.

The purpose of these studies was to assess the prevalence of psychiatric disorder in adult populations residing in the community so as to determine the full range of disorder and the proportion of people suffering from psychiatric disorder who were not receiving services. In total, over 20,000 individuals were included in the study, about 18,000 from the general population and about 2,500 from various institutionalized populations. People were interviewed using the National Institute of Mental Health Diagnostic Interview Schedule (DIS). The DIS is a highly structured interview that was administered by highly trained, lay interviewers. When computer analyzed, the DIS yields psychiatric diagnoses based on research diagnostic criteria embedded in the *Diagnostic and Statistical Manual of Mental Disorders* (DSM) of the American Psychiatric Association. It serves as a benchmark study for examining the prevalence of psychiatric disorders in the general population.

MAJOR ISSUES ADDRESSED IN THIS REVIEW

The following questions are examined in this review:

1. Does the prevalence of anxiety disorders differ among ethnic and cultural groups?
2. Do the risk factors for developing anxiety differ among ethnic and cultural groups?
3. What are the differences in symptom pattern of the expressions of anxiety across cultures?
4. What culture-specific syndromes and idioms of distress might fit, at least in part, within the anxiety disorders section of DSM-IV (4th edition of the DSM; American Psychiatric Association, 1994) and how do these cultural categories raise questions about the DSM diagnostic criteria?
5. Is the diagnosis of posttraumatic stress disorder appropriate for categorizing the experience of refugees from Southeast Asia and Central America and do the criteria for posttraumatic stress disorder need to be modified for these groups?
6. What contribution would the addition of a mixed anxiety–depression diagnosis make to incorporating cross-cultural expressions of anxiety?

Studies were selected for this chapter that (1) updated findings in the review by Good and Kleinman (1985), (2) focused on psychiatric diagnosis (i.e., for their assessment of anxiety disorders) rather than psychological assessment (i.e., anxiety as a continuous dimension), and (3) provided insights into the major anxiety disorders listed in DSM-IV.

PREVALENCE OF ANXIETY DISORDERS IN MULTICULTURAL SETTINGS

Two recent epidemiological reports of anxiety disorders using the ECA data indicate that there are important similarities and differences in the prevalence of selected anxiety disorders among different ethnic and cultural groups. Table 1.1 provides a summary of the rates of the major anxiety disorders among Mexican Americans and non-Hispanic whites

TABLE 1.1. Lifetime Prevalence of Selected Anxiety Disorders by Ethnicity

	Mexican American		Non-Hispanic whites
	Born in Mexico	Born in the United States	
Disorder	(N = 706)	(N = 538)	(N = 1,149)
OCD	1.6 (0.5)	2.4 (0.8)	3.2 (0.6)
Panic	1.2 (0.5)	1.0 (0.3)	1.9 (0.4)
GAD	2.9 (0.8)	5.1 (1.0)	10.0 (0.8)
Phobia			
Simple	7.8 (1.3)	12.7 (1.6)	6.8 (0.7)
Agoraphobia	4.7 (1.1)	7.6 (1.1)	3.9 (0.6)
Social	2.3 (0.8)	3.4 (0.8)	2.3 (0.5)

Note. Data from the Los Angeles ECA site (Karno et al., 1989, p. 206). Numbers in parentheses are standard errors. OCD, obsessive–compulsive disorder; GAD, generalized anxiety disorder.

in the Los Angeles ECA study. Table 1.2 compares the rates of lifetime and recent phobias between African Americans and whites in the Baltimore and St. Louis ECA sites.

In an analysis by Karno and colleagues (1989) of the prevalence of the full range of anxiety disorders in the Los Angeles ECA site, similar prevalences of panic disorder, social phobia, and obsessive–compulsive disorder were found when comparing non-Hispanic whites with Mexican Americans born either in the United States or in Mexico. Differences were found for the diagnoses of simple phobia, agoraphobia, and generalized anxiety disorder. A major finding of this study was that Mexicans born in Mexico had lower rates of anxiety (and other disorders) than Mexican Americans born in the United States. The authors suggest selective migration as a key factor in the differences in rates.

TABLE 1.2. Prevalence of Phobia by Ethnicity

	Baltimore		St. Louis	
	Black	White	Black	White
Disorder	(N = 1,182)	(N = 2,193)	(N = 1,158)	(N = 1743)
Simple (lifetime)	27.6	17.4	11.1	5.9
Agoraphobia (lifetime)	13.4	7.2		
Recent (1 month)	15.8	9.8	8.5	4.1

Note. Data from the Baltimore and St. Louis ECA sites (Brown et al., 1990, p. 437).

From the perspective of cross-cultural psychiatry, much research is needed to explore in detail the nature of the migration experience and of long-term residence in the urban United States to understand the source of these differences and to identify preventive interventions for the children of these immigrants.

A paper by Brown and colleagues (1990) reviews data on phobias from the Baltimore and St. Louis ECA sites, both sites with large numbers of African American respondents. The authors found that African Americans had higher rates of phobias than whites, even when sociodemographic factors were controlled. They suggested that greater numbers of stressful life events and higher stress from marginal minority group status (i.e., racism) may account for the higher rates of phobias among African Americans (p. 44). An analysis by Horwath, Johnson, and Hornig (1993) of the ECA data found considerable similarities between African American and European American subjects in their rates of panic disorder and patterns of panic symptoms.

The ECA studies suggest important ethnic differences, as well as similarities, in rates of anxiety disorders and offer hypotheses relating to different sociocultural experiences as explanations for these differences, as analyses demonstrated that social-class factors alone were not sufficient explanations. Yet measures of these social experiences of marginality and social stress are lacking in many epidemiological studies and are greatly needed to further mental health research generally and cross-cultural research in particular. None of the ECA studies raise the validity issue of using the anxiety questions, particularly the phobia questions, as measures of psychiatric disorder rather than as measures of social stresses. Considerable research is needed to establish whether elevated symptoms of anxiety, particularly phobia, are signs of a disordered individual or a disordered social environment.

A clinical study by Friedman and Paradis (1991), which compares 15 African American patients with panic and agoraphobia to 15 white patients with panic and agoraphobia, specifies some of the life events that may be related to higher rates of anxiety disorders among African Americans. Both groups with panic and agoraphobia had similar symptom profiles. The authors found that the African Americans with panic and agoraphobia experienced more separations from parents and more trauma events in childhood than the white patients. They also experienced worse treatment outcome.

Friedman and colleagues (1994) carried out a larger study to explore symptom presentations and treatment issues between African American and European American patients with panic disorder and agoraphobia. There were *no* significant differences across ethnic groups in the symptom profiles of the panic attacks. As in the earlier study,

African American patients were more likely to have experienced parental separations and to have a parental history of substance abuse. However, African American patients were less likely to have a parental history of anxiety or depression. Of particular interest for this cultural review is the significantly higher report of sleep paralysis by African American subjects in the study, both from clinical and community groups. Simons and Hughes, in their book *The Culture-Bound Syndromes* (1985), identify a sleep paralysis category of cultural syndromes with detailed case studies from Newfoundland, where it is labeled the "old hag" phenomenon (see also Hufford, 1982), and similar experiences among the Inuit in Alaska. More work is needed to identify particular cultural features of sleep paralysis among African Americans. Similarly, Friedman and colleagues note that some clinicians misdiagnose African American patients' concerns about "root work" (a practice among some African Americans, especially in the South, of using magical objects to harm or heal others) as psychosis rather than viewing it as anxiety about malign magic. This raises the more general point that severe worry about supernatural concerns across cultures (e.g., concerns about spirit possession, malign magic, fate, and bewitchment) are often misdiagnosed by European American clinicians as psychotic disorders because these kinds of experiences are "abnormal" within the dominant Anglo-American cultural context. However, these experiences with and concerns about the supernatural are quite common across the globe and do not necessarily represent serious thought disorders. Nevertheless, in some cases, disabling apprehension about such spiritual matters may be appropriately diagnosed within the framework of the anxiety disorders.

CROSS-CULTURAL DIFFERENCES IN PATTERNS OF ANXIETY SYMPTOMS

Although ethnic comparisons within the United States have not identified major symptom differences for the anxiety disorders, cross-cultural studies have indicated that there are significant differences in the ways anxiety is described, and potentially, experienced. A key implication of this work is that the range of symptoms included in DSM-IV may need to be expanded to make the manual applicable across cultures and that, in some cases, diagnostic criteria may also need to be modified. Of particular concern is the primary emphasis on the emotional experiences of excessive worry or apprehension as the key to diagnosis and the lack of emphasis on somatic forms or presentations of anxiety.

Many of the studies that have detailed the differential report of anxiety symptoms have come from Nigeria in West Africa, including clinical studies of both culture-specific syndromes (Makanjuola, 1987) and of anxiety (Awaritefe, 1988), and the development of the Enugu Somatization Scale by Ebigbo (1986). Several of the studies indicated that a core symptom of anxiety, as experienced in Nigeria, was a sensation of an insect or parasite crawling through the head and sometimes other parts of the body (Ebigbo, 1986; Makanjuola, 1987; Awaritefe, 1988). More broadly, these studies demonstrated that when symptoms were freely listed by those suffering anxiety and were systematically studied (see Ebigbo, 1986), new criterial symptoms emerged for the anxiety disorders. These studies call into question findings in the United States that symptom patterns are not significantly different among ethnic groups. Studies in the United States all used structured instruments that only allowed for response to a limited set of symptom items originally derived from European American populations, rather than starting by freely eliciting anxiety symptoms from a culturally diverse group of patients. In the next section, I will examine some cultural syndromes that relate to the anxiety disorders and highlight some of the key symptoms of these syndromes, which are not now fully described in the DSM-IV section on anxiety.

CULTURAL SYNDROMES AND THEIR RELATIONSHIP TO ANXIETY DISORDERS

A brief discussion of some culture-specific syndromes that have been proposed for inclusion within the anxiety disorders underscores the following issues: (1) the need for an expanded set of symptoms for the anxiety disorders; (2) the issue of the borderline between anxiety, affective, somatoform, and dissociative disorders; and (3) the need to expand the broader anxiety category to include cultural expressions that do not fit easily into existing anxiety diagnoses. Three syndromes that highlight these issues and about which there is considerable information, allowing comparison with DSM-IV diagnoses, include *ataques de nervios* (Guarnaccia, Rubio-Stipec, & Canino, 1989; Guarnaccia, Canino, Rubio-Stipec, & Bravo, 1993), *koro* (Bernstein & Gaw, 1990), and *taijin kyofusho* (Kirmayer, 1991).

Ataques de Nervios

I analyzed an epidemiological study of the mental health of Puerto Rican adults in Puerto Rico that included a question on *ataque de nervios*, a syndrome most widely studied among Puerto Ricans but also common among Caribbean Hispanics and reported in other areas of Latin America as well (Guarnaccia et al., 1993). In eliciting experiences of *ataques de nervios*, the most common symptom reported was "screaming uncontrollably," a symptom that does not appear in DSM-IV. "Attacks of crying" was the next most prominent symptom; it appears in the somatization section of the DIS and is most often associated with affective disorders. Although the symptom profile of an *ataque de nervios* is closest to a panic attack in DSM-IV, major differences between *ataques* and panic attacks include that (1) *ataques* are usually provoked by an upsetting event whereas panic attacks occur in situations that are not inherently upsetting or frightening and (2) the hallmark symptom, in panic attacks, of acute fear or apprehension of future attacks is frequently absent in *ataques de nervios*. In looking at the association between experiencing an *ataque de nervios* and meeting criteria for psychiatric disorders, we (Guarnaccia et al., 1989, 1993) found significant associations not only with anxiety but also with affective disorders. More recent work on the phenomenology of *ataques de nervios* (Guarnaccia, Rivera, Franco, & Neighbors, 1996) highlights a strong anger and loss of impulse control dimension to *ataques* as well as significant dissociative features such as fainting, loss of memory, and waking up in a new place (such as a hospital) without knowing how one got there. In current, unpublished analyses of data collected from people who had experienced an *ataque de nervios* using a structured diagnostic interview, it is the presence of these dissociative experiences that most closely correlate with a person with *ataques* meeting criteria for psychiatric disorder. For the clinician working with Puerto Rican and other Latino clients, reports of an *ataque de nervios* can be viewed as a risk marker for a range of anxiety, depressive, and dissociative disorders. Only by getting more detailed phenomenological descriptions of the *ataque*, its provoking events, and the psychological and emotional sequelae of the episode can clinicians determine the most appropriate diagnosis and treatment strategy for the individual.

Koro

The defining feature of *koro* is "acute anxiety associated with the fear of genital retraction and is usually accompanied by the thought that complete disappearance of the organ into the abdomen will result in death" (Bernstein & Gaw, 1990, p. 1670). It has been reported in several Asian cultural groups and has been described in both Eastern and Western medical texts for centuries. In proposing a DSM-IV classification for the syndrome, Bernstein and Gaw note the dilemmas of fitting *koro* into current diagnostic categories. Although acute anxiety is a core feature of the syndrome arguing for an anxiety disorder, the defining feature is concern over a physical symptom (genital retraction) with no physiological basis arguing for a somatoform disorder. Another key feature of *koro* is that it has occurred in both individual and large group manifestations. Again, clinicians working with Asian patients who experience these symptoms need to get a richer contextual picture of how the individual's experience is understood by and potentially shared with significant others and assess whether the predominant concerns are fear of the possibility of genital retraction or distorted perception of changes in the body. As in the example previously mentioned of mistaking supernatural concerns as psychosis; it is important in *koro* not to assume significant thought disorder unless the distortions in perception have persisted for an extensive period of time and led to significant functional impairment. Often the input of significant others from the family and cultural group about the content and nature of the experience is essential, as is true in much cross-cultural clinical work.

Taijin Kyofusho

Kirmayer (1991; Kirmayer et al., 1995) analyzes the fit of *taijin kyofusho* into DSM-IV criteria as part of a broader cultural critique of psychiatric diagnosis. *Taijin kyofusho* is a syndrome particular to Japan involving anxiety or fears that certain features of personal style or of one's physical self will give offense *to* others. *Taijin kyofusho* reverses the usual definitions of social phobia (anxiety of being scrutinized or embarrassed *by* others in social situations) found in DSM-IV. Kirmayer (1991, p. 21) notes that fear of blushing, fear of eye-to-eye contact, and fear of emitting body odor, all symptoms of *taijin kyofusho*, are symptoms that are absent from DSM-IV. Kirmayer argues that the different subtypes of *taijin kyofusho* described in Japanese psychiatry would range from adjustment disorders in childhood to delusional disorders in DSM-IV. Japanese psychiatry recognizes *taijin kyofusho* as a disorder, and Morita developed a particular form of indigenous psychotherapy specifically designed to deal with the problems of excessive self-awareness that underlie *taijin kyofusho* (Kirmayer et al., 1995).

POSTTRAUMATIC STRESS DISORDER IN REFUGEES

Posttraumatic stress disorder has received considerable recent attention from cross-cultural researchers in the United States and other places because of its applicability and high prevalence among refugee groups from Southeast Asia and Central America who are fleeing violence and state terror (Mollica, Wyshak, & Lavelle, 1987; Mollica et al., 1990; Eisenbruch, 1991; Jenkins, 1991). Although posttraumatic stress disorder is considered an anxiety disorder, clinicians and researchers working with these refugees have found a high co-occurrence of major depressive disorder (Kinzie et al., 1990; Mollica et al., 1987; Jenkins, 1991) and of dissociative experiences (Carlson & Rosser-Hogan, 1991) with posttraumatic stress disorder. Eisenbruch (1991) has proposed an alternative category of "cultural bereavement" for Southeast Asian refugees as a diagnosis that more fully captures the nature of the syndrome of traumatic losses experienced by refugees. The recency of the posttraumatic stress disorder diagnosis and its even more recent application to groups who are culturally different and whose trauma experience is unique suggest a need for considerable research before conclusions can be reached about the applicability of posttraumatic stress disorder to these populations or the place of posttraumatic stress disorder within the diagnostic system.

THE ROLE OF MIXED ANXIETY–DEPRESSION IN THE ANXIETY DISORDERS

Mixed anxiety–depression was proposed as a new disorder for the DSM-IV anxiety disorders. This disorder was seen as particularly needed for primary care settings where patients often presented a subsyndromal picture of anxiety and depression together. Cross-cultural researchers have also stressed the need for a mixed anxiety–depression diagnosis that would better fit with many cultural idioms of distress that cut across the borders of the anxiety, affective, and somatoform disorders. Also, mixed anxiety–depression is currently part of the International Classification of Diseases. The DSM-IV field trials (Zinbarg et al., 1994) included a Hispanic sample from the Hispanic Anxiety Clinic at the New York State Psychiatric Institute (Liebowitz et al., 1994) to test the reliability and validity of the diagnosis. Some of the preliminary findings from this field trial further highlight cross-cultural issues in the assessment of anxiety.

In the DSM-IV field trial of mixed anxiety–depression, 15–20% of Hispanic subjects received a not otherwise specified (NOS) diagnosis, making it the third most prominent diagnosis after generalized anxiety disorder and panic disorder. This was a much higher proportion than at the other sites, which consisted overwhelmingly of European American subjects. The conclusion of the researchers was that a significant proportion of the Hispanic subsample reported emotional disturbance not captured by the current diagnostic system. This NOS group would have fit into a mixed anxiety–depression diagnosis had it been recognized officially by the DSM-IV Task Force. In the anxiety NOS and generalized anxiety disorder groups in the Hispanic subsample, there was an emphasis on the somatic symptoms of anxiety. This contrasted with the broader field trial sample, which reported more negative affect than physiological arousal. Although 77% of the NOS cases reported at least one sphere of worry, in half of these cases neither the patient nor the clinician judged the worry to be excessive. The Hispanic subsample was the only subsample that was made up of predominantly poor, recently arrived immigrants with limited education and English ability. More explicitly comparative research efforts like this are clearly needed.

CULTURAL CONSIDERATIONS FOR THE ANXIETY DISORDERS

Based on the above review, the following recommendations of cultural features were suggested to include in the Anxiety Disorders section of DSM-IV. The recommendations are organized by diagnosis as was requested by the DSM-IV editorial committee.

Generalized Anxiety Disorder

Across cultures, there is a rich somatic vocabulary for the expression of anxiety that complements the expression of anxiety in emotional terms, such as excessive worry or apprehension. In applying generalized anxiety diagnostic criteria cross-culturally, attention needs to be given to the preponderance of concern with somatic symptoms and the expression of anxiety in bodily idioms of distress.

Panic Disorder

Understanding the social and cultural context of anxiety reactions may be critically important in making accurate diagnoses. Cultural syndromes may not be viewed as a disorder within the cultural context; the validity of referral and treatment of such cases in the psychiatric setting needs to be judged on a case-by-case basis with appropriate cultural consultation. In diagnosing panic disorder, the clinician must judge whether an anxiety reaction is unprovoked or is a response to a stressful event.

Agoraphobia

Some cultural and ethnic groups prescribe much more circumscribed public roles for members of the group, particularly women, than is common in American society. These restrictions on participation in public life may complicate the assessment of agoraphobia. The clinician will need to ascertain whether the fear of being in public is due to social sanctions or ostracism or whether the fear is an intrinsic fear of leaving the home or having a panic attack. This point is further supported by a study carried out by El-Islam in Qatar (cited in Kirmayer et al., 1995, p. 507). He found that only 8% of women in Qatar with phobias reported agoraphobia. El-Islam states, "Being bound to the home, which is a sign of severe agoraphobia in the West, is a sign of virtue in a Muslim housewife."

Specific Phobia and Social Phobia

Assessments of the excessiveness of fears, worries or concerns about the dangerousness of situations or objects will need to be made within the cultural context of the individual's reference group. The content of phobias as well as their prevalence varies with culture and ethnicity. Many important phobic responses in other cultural groups may not be contained in DSM-IV or may present differently across cultures. Two examples follow:

1. *Specific phobia.* Apprehension or vigilance toward a culturally salient fear of malign magic or spirits or a concern with being possessed or bewitched should be seen, in many cases, as symptomatic of anxiety rather than as a sign of a thought disorder.
2. *Social phobia.* The social phobia definition should be expanded to include concern about giving offense to others in social situations, such as the irrational fear that one's glance or body odor is offensive; that is, *taijin kyofusho* should be included in DSM-IV.

Obsessive–Compulsive Disorder

In societies where the regular performance of both public and private ritual are more central than in U.S. society, the definition of obsessive–compulsive disorder may be complicated because it is crucial to assess when the ritual behavior has become pathological. Important life transitions, rules about protecting oneself from "pollution," and mourning observances may lead to an intensification of ritual behavior that may appear to be obsessive to a clinician who is not familiar with the cultural context. Ritual behavior is not in itself indicative of obsessive–compulsive disorder unless it exceeds cultural norms, occurring at times and places judged inappropriate by others and interfering with social role functions. Clinicians may need to seek cultural guidance in how to assess whether behavior violates cultural norms. A recent article by Dulaney and Fiske (1994) provides a comparison of ritual behaviors from a wide range of cultures and of compulsions identified in psychiatric texts. They find considerable parallel between the specific behaviors carried out during rituals and by people with obsessive–compulsive disorder, though marked differences in the motivations. In rituals, these behaviors are part of a cultural meaning system that brings order to the world; in obsessive–compulsive disorder, the behaviors are invented in isolation, with meanings that do not make sense to the community, and are regarded as bizarre and of doubtful efficacy by others and often by the patient. "It is this meaninglessness and incompatibility, not the morphology of the actions or the content of the thoughts, that constitutes OCD, [obsessive–compulsive disorder]" (pp. 247–248). The implications of their article further our concern that cross-cultural application of this category may be more complex than many clinicians appreciate.

Posttraumatic Stress Disorder

For recent migrants coming from areas of considerable social unrest and civil conflict, the diagnosis of posttraumatic stress disorder should be considered when the person reports significant somatic and/or psychological distress. Of particular note are symptoms of sleep troubles and frightening dreams. Considerable experience with refugees from Southeast Asia and Central America indicate that traumatic experiences of violence and state terror are widespread among refugees from these areas. Specific assessments of traumatic experiences are needed for these groups. Depending on the nature of the trauma and the symptoms, differential diagnosis will focus on determining whether anxiety, depression, or dissociation is the more prominent feature of the syndrome.

DISCUSSION

The issues discussed above highlight major concerns about the cross-cultural applicability of the Anxiety Disorders section of DSM-IV and raise challenges for DSM-IV. The current lists of criterial symptoms in

DSM-IV are a limited palette of the cross-cultural experience of anxiety. Some cultural syndromes may fit within the anxiety disorders with some modification of criteria or additions of subcategories. Many of the cultural syndromes raise a challenge to the current nosology, which separates the anxiety disorders from affective and somatoform disorders. Rather, a more interactive and integrated view of these disorders is required, which only begins to be addressed by the mixed anxiety–depression category that was proposed for DSM-IV.

Both psychiatric researchers and clinicians need to develop a more complex understanding of culture and its relationship to the expression of emotion and experience of disorder. Culture serves as the web that structures human thought, emotion, and interaction. Culture provides a variety of resources for dealing with major life changes and challenges, including serious illness and hospitalization. Culture is continuously being shaped by social processes such as migration and acculturation. Cultures vary not only by national, regional, or ethnic background, but by age, gender, and social class. Much of culture is embedded in and communicated by language, thus, language cannot be understood or used outside of its cultural context. Cross-cultural psychiatric and medical anthropological research focuses on the role of culture in shaping expressions of distress, in this case, on various ways of experiencing and expressing forms of anxiety. This research literature can be very valuable to clinicians working in a multicultural society. Clinicians also need to learn about these various cultural dimensions of their clients so as to interpret and contextualize more accurately the concerns and symptoms their clients bring to them. At the same time, clinicians who carefully assess and document their clients' expressions and experiences can continue to inform the research community about the varieties of anxiety and their expressions. This review of cross-cultural literature has focused more on assessment issues than treatment because of the centrality of understanding the nature of a client's problem in the initial phase of treating them. Clinicians can further contribute to our cross-cultural understanding by documenting the differences these kinds of careful, culturally informed assessments make in treatment selection and the outcomes of different therapeutic interventions.

RECOMMENDATIONS

In light of the above comments, the following recommendations are made for the continuing examination of cross-cultural issues in the anxiety disorders:

1. More systematic research is needed to identify the range of symptoms prominently associated with anxiety disorders in different cultural groups and different cultural contexts.
2. For those cultural syndromes about which we have considerable detailed information from clinical and/or epidemiological research, multidisciplinary research efforts between psychiatric and cross-cultural researchers are needed to assess the relationship of these syndromes with current diagnostic categories and the need for new subcategories or categories of disorder.
3. For cultural syndromes where the level of knowledge is currently insufficient to assess their relationship to psychiatric categories, research efforts are needed to describe and assess more fully these idioms of distress and their impact on those who suffer from them.
4. Recognition of the interplay among the anxiety, affective, somatoform, and dissociative disorders is needed to open the possibility for research that would examine the appropriateness of these categorizations and the place of cultural forms of expressing distress and cultural syndromes within them.
5. It would be very useful to have guidelines for clinicians in obtaining cultural consultation on the issues raised in this review. Valuable initiatives include the development of a cultural casebook and the design of specific training for mental health professionals, both during graduate study and as part of continuing professional education.

REFERENCES

American Psychiatric Association. (1994). *Diagnostic and statistical manual of mental disorders* (4th ed.). Washington, DC: Author..

Awaritefe, A. (1988). Clinical anxiety in Nigeria. *Acta Psychiatrica Scandinavica, 77,* 729–735.

Bernstein, R. L., & Gaw, A. C. (1990). Koro: Proposed classification for DSM-IV. *American Journal of Psychiatry, 147,* 1670–1674.

Brown, D. R., Eaton, W. W., & Sussman, L. (1990). Racial differences in prevalence of phobic disorders. *Journal of Nervous and Mental Disease, 178,* 434–441.

Carlson, E. B., & Rosser-Hogan, R. (1991). Trauma experiences, posttraumatic stress, dissociation, and depression in Cambodian refugees. *American Journal of Psychiatry, 148,* 1548–1551.

Dulaney, S., & Fiske, A. P. (1994). Cultural rituals and obsessive–compulsive disorder: Is there a common psychological mechanism? *Ethos, 22,* 243–283.

Ebigbo, P. O. (1986). A cross sectional study of somatic complaints of Nigerian females using the Enugu Somatization Scale. *Culture, Medicine and Psychiatry, 10,* 167–186.

Eisenbruch, M. (1991). From post-traumatic stress disorder to cultural bereavement: Diagnosis of Southeast Asian Refugees. *Social Science and Medicine, 33,* 673–680.

Friedman, S., & Paradis, C. (1991). African-American patients with panic disorder and agoraphobia. *Journal of Anxiety Disorders, 5,* 35–41.

Friedman, S., Paradis, C. M., & Hatch, M. (1994). Characteristics of African American and white patients with panic disorder and agoraphobia. *Hospital and Community Psychiatry, 45,* 798–803.

Good, B. J., & Kleinman, A. M. (1985). Culture and anxiety: Cross-cultural evidence for the patterning of anxiety disorders. In A. H. Tuma & J. Maser (Eds.), *Anxiety and the anxiety disorders* (pp. 297–324). Hillsdale, NJ: Erlbaum.

Guarnaccia, P. J., Canino, G., Rubio-Stipec, M., & Bravo, M. (1993). The prevalence of ataques de nervios in the Puerto Rico Disaster Study. *Journal of Nervous and Mental Disease, 181,* 157–165.

Guarnaccia, P. J., & Kirmayer, L. J. (1997). Culture and the anxiety disorders. In T. A. Widiger, A. Frances, H. A. Pincus, R. Ross, M. B. First, & W. Davis (Eds.), *DSM-IV Sourcebook* (Vol. 3, pp. 925–932). Washington, DC: American Psychiatric Association.

Guarnaccia, P. J., Rivera, M., Franco, F., & Neighbors, C. (1996). The experiences of ataques de nervios: Towards an anthropology of emotions in Puerto Rico. *Culture, Medicine and Psychiatry, 20*(3), 343–367.

Guarnaccia, P. J., Rubio-Stipec, M., & Canino, G. (1989). Ataques de nervios in the Puerto Rican Diagnostic Interview Schedule. *Culture, Medicine and Psychiatry, 13,* 275–295.

Horwath, E., Johnson, J., & Hornig, C. D. (1993). Epidemiology of panic disorder in African Americans. *American Journal of Psychiatry, 150,* 465–468.

Hufford, D. C. (1982). *The terror that comes in the night.* Philadelphia: University of Pennsylvania Press.

Jenkins, J. H. (1991). The state construction of affect: Political ethos and mental health among Salvadoran refugees. *Culture, Medicine and Psychiatry, 15,* 139–165.

Karno, M., Golding, J. M., Burnham, M. A., Hough, R. L., Escobar, J. I., Wells, K. M., & Boyer, R. (1989). Anxiety disorders among Mexican Americans and non-Hispanic whites in Los Angeles. *Journal of Nervous and Mental Disease, 177,* 202–209.

Kinzie, J. D., Boehnlein, J. K., Leung, P. K., Moore, L. J., Riley, C., & Smith, D. (1990). The prevalence of posttraumatic stress disorder and its clinical significance among Southeast Asian refugees. *American Journal of Psychiatry, 147,* 913–917.

Kirmayer, L. J. (1991). The place of culture in psychiatric nosology: Taijin kyofusho and DSM-III-R. *Journal of Nervous and Mental Disease, 179,* 19–28.

Kirmayer, L. J., Young, A., & Hayton, B. C. (1995). The cultural context of anxiety disorders. In R. D. Alarcon (Ed.), *The psychiatric clinics of North America,* (pp. 503–521*).* Philadelphia: Saunders.

Liebowitz, M. R., Salman, E., Jusino, C. J., Garfinkel, R., Street, L., Cardenas, D. L., Silvestre, J., Fyer, A., Carrasco, J. L., Davies, S., Guarnaccia, P., & Klein, D. F. (1994). Ataque de nervios and panic disorder. *American Journal of Psychiatry, 151,* 871–875.

Makanjuola, R. O. A. (1987). "Ode Ori": A culture-bound disorder with prominent somatic features in Yoruba Nigerian patients. *Acta Psychiatrica Scandinavica, 75,* 231–236.

Mollica, R. F., Wyshak, G., & Lavelle, J. (1987). The psychosocial impact of war trauma and torture on Southeast Asian refugees. *American Journal of Psychiatry, 144,* 1567–1572.

Mollica, R. F., Wyshak, G., Lavelle, J., Truong, T., Tor, S., & Yang, T. (1990). Assessing symptom change in Southeast Asian refugee survivors of mass violence and torture. *American Journal of Psychiatry, 147,* 83–88.

Regier, D. A., Myers, J. K., Kramer, M., Robins, L. N., Blazer, D. G., Hough, R. L., Eaton, W. W., & Locke, B. Z. (1984). The NIMH Epidemiologic Catchment Area program. *Archives of General Psychiatry, 41,* 934–941.

Simons, R. C., & Hughes, C. C. (1985). *The culture-bound syndromes.* Dordrecht, The Netherlands: Reidel.

World Health Organization. (1973). *The International Pilot Study of Schizophrenia.* Geneva: Author.

World Health Organization. (1979). *Schizophrenia: An international follow-up study.* Chichester, UK: Wiley.

World Health Organization. (1983). *Depressive disorders in different cultures.* Geneva: Author.

Zinbarg, R. E., Barlow, D. H., Liebowitz, M. R., Street, L. L., Broadhead, E., Katon, W., Roy-Byrne, P., Lepine, J., Teherani, M., Richards, J., Brantley, P., & Kraemer, H. (1994). The DSM-IV field trial for mixed anxiety–depression. *American Journal of Psychiatry, 151,* 1153–1162.

2

Epidemiology of Anxiety Disorders across Cultural Groups

EWALD HORWATH
MYRNA M. WEISSMAN

Anxiety has been recognized as a symptom ever since the writings of Freud. However, it was only recently, with the incorporation into the third edition of the *Diagnostic and Statistical Manual of Mental Disorders* (DSM-III) and DSM-III-R (revised) (American Psychiatric Association, 1980, 1987) of Klein's conceptualization of panic disorder as a separate entity, that anxiety states began to be subdivided into distinct disorders such as panic, phobias, generalized anxiety disorder, and obsessive–compulsive disorder. Cross-cultural investigation of prevalence rates suggests that the anxiety disorders may have differential distribution across racial, gender, and cultural boundaries.

In a review of five population studies conducted in the United States, the United Kingdom, and Sweden prior to the development of specified diagnostic criteria, Marks and Lader (1973) found that anxiety states were fairly common (about 2.0–4.7/100 point prevalence) and were more prevalent in women, particularly younger women between 16 and 40 years of age. In a separate epidemiological review, Weissman (1985) identified nine additional community studies of anxiety states that showed rates in the range reported by Marks and Lader (1973), and also showed that rates were higher in women than in men. Our focus in this chapter is on the more recent epidemiological studies in which anxiety disorders are subdivided on the basis of DSM-III or DSM-III-R criteria (Eaton, Dryman, & Weissman,1991; Weissman et al., 1988; Bland, Newman, & Orn, 1988; Canino et al., 1987; Faravelli, Degl'Innocenti, & Giardinelli, 1989; Lee, Han, & Choi, 1987; Lee et al., 1990a, 1990b; Hwu, Yeh, & Chang, 1989; Joyce, Bushnell, Oakley-Brown, Wells, & Hornblow, 1989; Angst & Dobler-Mikola, 1985).

EPIDEMIOLOGICAL APPROACH
TO CROSS-CULTURAL QUESTIONS

The epidemiological approach to the cross-cultural study of anxiety disorders is associated with certain strengths and weaknesses. Epidemiological studies are very informative because they gather data from large numbers of subjects, use powerful statistical techniques, and survey community samples of people who are not in treatment. The study of large numbers of subjects allows for comparisons across relevant groups based on differences in gender, race, education, occupation, ethnicity, and other cultural and socioeconomic factors. Large numbers also provide the statistical power to use sophisticated analytic strategies, such as multivariate regression analysis, which can dissect the effects of complex sociodemographic variables. Community surveys can sample nonclinical populations, which allows the investigation of cultural variables without the confounding factor of treatment seeking, which is strongly influenced by cultural factors.

Epidemiological studies also have limitations in their capacity to answer cross-cultural questions regarding psychiatric disorders. First, "culture" is a complex concept that has not been clearly defined for purposes of epidemiological study. Sociodemographic variables, such as gender, race, education, ethnicity, language, and religion, are measured in epidemiological surveys in an attempt to capture some of what is meant by the term "culture." However, some of the more subtle aspects of culture, such as an individual's sense of origin or important values, may have powerful influences on psychiatric symptom formation, but are not easily measured in a large community survey. Finally, the diagnostic constructs used in epidemiological surveys may be well established in industrially developed, Western societies, but their reliability and validity may not be adequately tested across other cultures.

PANIC DISORDER

Definition

The key feature of panic disorder in DSM-III is the occurrence of three or more panic attacks within a 3-week period. These attacks cannot be precipitated only by exposure to a feared situation, cannot be due to a physical disorder, and must be accompanied by at least four of the following symptoms: dyspnea, palpitations, chest pain, smothering or choking, dizziness, feelings of unreality, paresthesia, hot and cold flashes, sweating, faintness, trembling, or shaking (American Psychiatric Association, 1980). In DSM-III-R, the definition was revised to require four attacks in 4 weeks or one or more attacks followed by a persistent fear of having another attack, and the list of potential symptoms was revised to include nausea or abdominal distress and to exclude depersonalization or derealization (American Psychiatric Association, 1987).

More importantly, DSM-III-R changed the diagnostic hierarchy so that panic disorder could be diagnosed as a primary disorder with or without agoraphobia, and dropped the category of agoraphobia with panic attacks. This change placed the emphasis on identifying panic disorder as a discrete entity and reflected the clinical experience that panic attacks tended to occur prior to the development of agoraphobia, which was increasingly viewed as a phobic avoidance response to the frightening experience of spontaneous panic attacks, near panic experiences, or limited symptom attacks.

Rates

Table 2.1 shows prevalence rates of panic disorder from community studies using DSM-III or DSM-III-R criteria. For studies using DSM-III, the 6-month prevalence of panic disorder ranged from 0.6/100 in New Haven, Connecticut, to 1.1/100 in Puerto Rico, representing a remarkable level of consistency across sites. The annual prevalence rate of 3.1/100 from the Zurich survey was based on a definition of panic that only approximated that of DSM-III. The National Comorbidity Study (NCS) reported a 1-year prevalence of 2.3/100 for DSM-III-R panic disorder (Kessler, McGonagle, Zhao, Nelson, Hughes, Eshleman, Wittchen, & Kendler, 1994).

Lifetime rates of DSM-III panic disorder showed good agreement, with prevalence varying from 1.2/100 in Edmonton, Canada, to 2.2/100 in New Zealand. The exception to this narrow range of lifetime rates was Taiwan, where panic disorder occurred at rates from 0.13/100

TABLE 2.1. Prevalence Rates per 100 of Panic Disorder Using DSM-III (or DSM-III-R) Criteria

Place	Rate/100		
	6-month	1-year	Lifetime
United States: NCS (DSM-III-R)		2.3	3.5
United States: ECA (five sites)			1.6
New Haven, CT	0.6		
Baltimore, MD	1.0		
St. Louis, MO	0.9		
Piedmont, NC	0.7		
Los Angeles, CA	0.9		
Zurich, Switzerland		3.1	
Edmonton, Canada	0.7		1.2
Puerto Rico	1.1		1.7
New Zealand			2.2
Florence, Italy			1.4
Korea			1.7
Taiwan			
Urban			0.20
Small towns			0.34
Rural			0.13

Note. Adapted from Horwath and Weissman (1995). Copyright 1995 by Wiley-Liss. Adapted by permission.

in rural areas to 0.34/100 in small towns. The only study that reported on lifetime DSM-III-R panic disorder was the NCS, which found a rate of 3.5/100, considerably higher than the lifetime rates based on DSM-III. This may be due to the broadening of the concept of panic disorder in DSM-III-R or to the differences in memory probes used in the NCS University of Michigan version of the Composite International Diagnostic Interview (UM-CIDI), as compared to those used in the Diagnostic Interview Schedule (DIS).

Risk Factors

Sex

Comparing lifetime prevalence rates, all of the studies reporting on panic disorder showed higher rates for women than for men. With the exception of Puerto Rico and Taiwan, the higher lifetime risk for women was statistically significant in all of the community studies. In an analysis of the NCS data, Eaton, Kessler, Wittchen, and Magee (1994) found uniformly higher rates of panic attacks and panic disorder for women compared to men within every age group. Keyl and Eaton (1990) analyzed incidence rates from the Epidemiologic Catchment

Area (ECA) study and found a two-fold increased risk of incident panic disorder in women compared to men. This finding is analogous to the increased incidence and prevalence rates for major depression in women compared to men, and suggests that for both panic disorder and major depression the higher rates in women reflect a true increase in the risk for new onset panic and depression rather than a greater tendency to seek treatment or have longer episodes of illness.

Age

In both the NCS and the ECA data, a bimodal distribution of age of onset was reported (Eaton et al., 1994; Anthony & Aboraya, 1992). The NCS found an early mode for panic disorder in the age range of 15–24 years for both men and women, and a later mode in the 45–54 range (Eaton et al., 1994).

In the ECA and Edmonton studies, older persons (65 and over) had the lowest lifetime prevalence rates of panic disorder. This pattern was quite different for Hispanics in the ECA and Puerto Rican studies (Karno et al., 1987; Canino et al., 1987). In Puerto Rico and in Hispanic women in the ECA, the lifetime prevalence tended to increase with age. For Hispanic men in the ECA, the lifetime rate dropped with each age group, reaching zero in the group over 65 years of age. The NCS reported no significant ethnic differences for young adults, but did find lower rates in nonwhite compared to white older age groups. The reason for these differences is not clear.

Race/Ethnicity

In the ECA study, there were no significant differences in prevalence rates between African American, Hispanic, and white groups (Horwath, Johnson, & Hornig, 1993; Eaton et al., 1991). Similarly, the NCS found no main effects of race/ethnicity, but did report an age-by-race/ethnicity interaction effect (see above). Comparisons of other studies are more remarkable for the cross-cultural similarities in rates of panic disorder, with the exception of the Taiwan study, which had substantially lower rates of panic. As with major depression, Korean prevalence rates of panic disorder were comparable to those in the West, whereas Taiwan's were much lower.

Summary

The prevalence of panic disorder was fairly uniform, with higher risks for women and persons under the age of 65. The NCS and ECA data suggested a bimodal distribution in the ages of onset. As with other disorders, the NCS reported higher lifetime rates whereas Taiwan found much lower rates of panic disorder.

AGORAPHOBIA

Definition

DSM-III agoraphobia is defined as a fear and avoidance of being in places or situations from which escape might be difficult or in which help might not be available in the event of sudden incapacitation (American Psychiatric Association, 1980). As a result of such fears, the agoraphobic person avoids travel outside the home or requires the accompaniment of a companion when away from home. Moderate cases may cause some constriction in lifestyle, whereas severe cases of agoraphobia may result in the person being completely housebound or unable to leave home unaccompanied.

As outlined in the Panic Disorder section above, DSM-III-R revised the diagnosis of agoraphobia to a condition accompanying panic disorder (panic disorder with agoraphobia). Although the diagnosis of agoraphobia without history of panic disorder was retained, this category emphasized the avoidance behavior as a response to the sudden development of anxiety or somatic symptoms (American Psychiatric Association, 1987). DSM-IV has further emphasized that the agoraphobic avoidance behavior occurs specifically in response to unexpected or situationally predisposed panic attacks or panic-like symptoms (American Psychiatric Association, 1994).

Rates

Table 2.2 shows prevalence rates of agoraphobia from community studies using DSM-III or DSM-III-R criteria. In the ECA study, 6-month prevalence rates ranged from 2.7/100 in St. Louis to 5.8/100 in Baltimore. Lifetime rates of agoraphobia showed considerable variation, from a low of 1.1/100 in urban Taiwan to a high of 6.9/100 in Puerto Rico. Some of this variation may have been due to the use of a translated DIS (Robins, Helzer, Croughan, & Ratcliff, 1981). If one considers only the studies carried out in primarily English-speaking countries, the lifetime prevalence rates vary over a narrower range, from 2.9/100 in Edmonton, Canada, to 5.6/100 in the ECA data from four sites. In spite of the changes in the diagnostic definition between DSM-III and DSM-III-R, the lifetime rates from the ECA and NCS studies (5.6 vs. 5.3/100, respectively) show remarkable consistency.

TABLE 2.2. Prevalence Rates per 100 of Agoraphobia Using DSM-III (or DSM-III-R) Criteria

Place	Rate/100[a]		
	6-month	1-year	Lifetime
United States: NCS (DSM-III-R)		2.8	5.3
United States: ECA (five sites)			5.6
New Haven, CT	2.8		
Baltimore, MD	5.8		
St. Louis, MO	2.7		
Piedmont, NC	5.4		
Los Angeles, CA	3.2		
Puerto Rico	3.9		6.9
Zurich, Switzerland	2.5		
New Zealand			3.8
Florence, Italy			1.3
Edmonton, Canada			2.9
Korea			2.7
Taiwan			
Urban			1.1
Small towns			1.5
Rural			1.3

Note. Adapted from Horwath and Weissman (1995). Copyright 1995 by Wiley-Liss. Adapted by permission.
[a]Panic with agoraphobia.

Risk Factors

Lifetime rates of agoraphobia were significantly higher for women than for men in each of the community studies. This is consistent with the gender differences found for panic disorder and major depression.

In the ECA study, lifetime prevalence of agoraphobia was higher among African Americans than among whites or Hispanics. The effects of race/ethnicity and gender combined to produce a considerable range in lifetime prevalence, from 2.9/100 in white males to 12/100 in African American women (Eaton et al., 1991). In the NCS, current agoraphobia (past month) was associated with an increased risk in African Americans compared to whites, and in homemakers compared to those working outside the home (Magee, Eaton, Wittchen, McGonagle, & Kessler, 1996). Current agoraphobia was inversely related to income and education in a bivariate analysis of the NCS data (Magee et al., 1996).

Two studies reported significant urban–rural differences in rates of agoraphobia, but they were in opposite directions. In Puerto Rico, a significantly higher lifetime prevalence was found in the urban area, whereas in Korea, the rural rate was higher. The NCS found no significant urban–rural differences in rates of agoraphobia.

Relationship between Agoraphobia and Panic

In DSM-III, agoraphobia was considered a separate phobic disorder that may or may not be accompanied by panic attacks. Largely due to the influence of Klein's (1981) argument that agoraphobia is a conditioned avoidance response to the aversive stimulus of spontaneous panic attacks, the diagnostic view of agoraphobia changed considerably in DSM-III-R, in which panic disorder is viewed as primary, with or without the secondary development of agoraphobia. An important factor in this change was the observation by Klein and others that, in clinic settings, agoraphobia rarely occurs without preceding spontaneous panic attacks or limited symptom attacks.

Considerable controversy continues regarding the nature of the relationship between agoraphobic avoidance and panic attacks. Marks (1987) and other European investigators have questioned the temporal precedence and causal role of panic attacks in the development of agoraphobia.

Contributing to the controversy are the large differences between clinical and community studies in their estimates of the relative prevalence of agoraphobia with and without panic attacks. Table 2.3 shows the results of published community and clinical studies that have reported data permitting calculation of the proportion of agoraphobics with a history of panic attacks.

The community-based surveys found that a substantial proportion of subjects with agoraphobia reported no history of panic attacks. In these studies, 80% of the subjects were interviewed by lay persons using the DIS. In contrast, clinic-based studies, using less structured interviews administered by clinicians, almost invariably found much lower rates of agoraphobia without panic.

Several explanations for this discrepancy have been suggested. One explanation is that samples of treated persons with any illness have higher rates of comorbidity than samples of untreated persons (Berkson, 1946). An alternative explanation is that community studies may have overestimated the rate of agoraphobia without panic disorder.

In a reanalysis of the ECA data on agoraphobia without panic (Horwath, Lish, Johnson, Hornig, & Weissman, 1993), 22 community cases of agoraphobia without panic were clinically reappraised and only a single case of probable agoraphobia without panic was found. The diagnostic reappraisal found that 19 (87%) of the cases had simple or social phobias rather than agoraphobia, or had no DSM-III phobia at all. The reappraisal also identified six cases of panic disorder, panic attacks, or limited symptom attacks that had been missed by the DIS interview. The authors concluded that community studies using the

TABLE 2.3. Reported Frequency of Agoraphobia without Panic Attacks

Author	Date	No. of agoraphobics w/o panic attacks	Total No. of agoraphobics	%
Community studies				
Thompson	1989[a]	88	104	85
Angst & Dobler-Mikola	1985	15	22	68
ECA		656	961	68
Wittchen	1986	13	26	50
Joyce et al.	1989	35[b]	76	46
Faravelli et al.	1989	4	14	29
Clinical studies				
Torgersen	1983[c]	8	26	31
Thyer & Himle	1985	20[d]	115	17
Argyle & Roth	1986	5	42	12
Garvey & Tuason	1984	1	13	8
Aronson & Logue	1987	2	36	6
Pollard, Bronson, & Kenney	1989	61[e]	993	6
Uhde et al.	1985	1	32	3
Barlow	1988	1[f]	42	2
DiNardo	1983	0	23	0
Breier	1986	0	54	0
Noyes	1986	0	67	0
Kleiner	1987	0	50	0
Thyer, Parrish, Curtis, Nesse, & Cameron	1985b	0	28	0

Note. Adapted from Horwath, Lish, Johnson, Hornig, and Weissman (1993). Copyright 1993 by the American Psychiatric Association. Adapted by permission.

[a]Reported on agoraphobia without panic disorder.

[b]10 of 35 subjects reported limited symptom attacks.

[c]Reported on agoraphobia without panic disorder.

[d]These subjects "often suffered from unpredictable somatic symptoms . . . functional equivalent to panic attacks."

[e]Some subjects had limited symptom attacks.

[f]Subject had limited symptom attacks.

DIS may have overestimated the prevalence of agoraphobia without panic attacks in the community. Similar to the ECA, an initial analysis of the NCS data found that only about one third of NCS agoraphobics reported a history of a panic attack. More detailed analyses of the NCS data are underway to determine whether agoraphobia without panic is in fact as common as the initial analyses suggest (Magee et al., 1996).

Summary

Prevalence rates of agoraphobia based on the DIS and DSM-III varied considerably. These rates and their variations by study are difficult to interpret for two reasons. First, the diagnostic view of agoraphobia has changed considerably since these studies were done. Second, a clinical reappraisal study of ECA cases of agoraphobia without panic attacks suggested that studies using the DIS may have overestimated rates of agoraphobia without panic. This overestimate may have been due to missed cases of panic disorder, panic attacks, and limited symptom attacks; and to difficulty differentiating the boundary between agoraphobia and simple phobias.

In spite of the problems suggested above, the community studies consistently found higher rates of agoraphobia among women than men, and the ECA and NCS studies found higher rates among African Americans than among whites.

SOCIAL PHOBIA

Definition

The central feature of DSM-III social phobia is a persistent, irrational fear accompanied by a compelling desire to avoid situations in which the subject may act in a humiliating or embarrassing way while under the scrutiny of others (American Psychiatric Association, 1980). DSM-III-R allowed for the phobic situation to be avoided or endured with intense anxiety, and added the requirement that the avoidant behavior interferes with occupational or social functioning or that there is marked distress about having the fear (American Psychiatric Association, 1987). Common social phobias involve fears of speaking or eating in public, urinating in public lavatories, writing in front of others, or saying foolish things in social situations.

Rates

Table 2.4 shows the lifetime prevalence of social phobia from studies using DSM-III or DSM-III-R criteria. Lifetime rates of DSM-III social phobia varied considerably, with a low of 0.4/100 in rural Taiwan and a high of 3.9/100 in New Zealand. It is not clear whether these contrasting rates reflect true cross-cultural differences or are due to differences in methodology or translation of the DIS. The lifetime prevalence rates of social phobia vary over a somewhat narrower range—from 1.7/100 in Edmonton, Canada, to 3.9/100 in New Zealand—when comparing rates from English-speaking countries.

TABLE 2.4. Lifetime Prevalence Rates per 100 of Social
Phobia Using DSM-III (or DSM-III-R) Criteria

Place	Rates/100
United States: NCS (DSM-III-R)	13.3
United States: ECA (four sites)	2.4
Baltimore, MD	3.1
St. Louis, MO	1.9
Durham, NC	3.2
Los Angeles, CA	1.8
Edmonton, Canada	1.7
Puerto Rico	1.6
New Zealand	3.9
Florence, Italy	1.0
Korea	0.6
Taiwan	
Urban	0.6
Small towns	0.5
Rural	0.4

Note. Adapted from Horwath and Weissman (1995). Copyright
1995 by Wiley-Liss. Adapted by permission.

The rate of lifetime DSM-III-R social phobia from the NCS was considerably higher (13.3/100) than in any of the DSM-III studies. Magee
and colleagues (1996) attributed the higher prevalence to differences between the DIS and UM-CIDI. The UM-CIDI uses a stem question based
on the broader DSM-III-R criteria allowing either avoidance of a feared
situation or endurance with intense anxiety, and it also asks about six
specific social-phobic fears (compared to three in the DIS), including the
high prevalence fears of using a public toilet, writing in front of others,
or talking to people and sounding foolish or having nothing to say.

Risk Factors

In an analysis of the ECA data from four sites (the New Haven site
used a version of the DIS that did not include social-phobia items),
Schneier, Johnson, Hornig, Liebowitz, and Weissman (1992) found that
lifetime prevalence rates of social phobia were highest among women
and persons who were younger (age 18–29 years), less educated, single,
and of lower socioeconomic class. In the NCS, higher rates were found
in women, students, those with less education or income, those who
never married, and those who live with their parents (Magee et al.,
1996). A significantly higher prevalence of lifetime social phobia was
also found among women in Korea and urban Taiwan, while no
significant gender differences were found in Edmonton, Puerto Rico,
or small town or rural areas of Taiwan.

GENERALIZED ANXIETY DISORDER

Definition

The DSM-III criteria for generalized anxiety disorder require the presence of unrealistic or excessive anxiety and worry, accompanied by symptoms from three of four categories: (1) motor tension, (2) autonomic hyperactivity, (3) vigilance and scanning, and (4) apprehensive expectation. The anxious mood must continue for at least a month, and the diagnosis is not made if phobias, panic disorder, or obsessive–compulsive disorder are present, or if the disturbance is due to another physical or mental disorder, such as hyperthyroidism, major depression, or schizophrenia (American Psychiatric Association, 1980). By this definition, generalized anxiety disorder is treated primarily as a residual category after the exclusion of the other major anxiety disorders. DSM-III-R narrowed the definition further by requiring a minimum of six symptoms and a duration of 6 months (American Psychiatric Association, 1987).

Rates

Table 2.5 shows the prevalence of generalized anxiety disorder from community studies using DSM-III or DSM-III-R criteria. In the ECA study, hierarchical diagnostic exclusion of panic disorder and major depression yielded the 1-year prevalence of 2.7/100, while dropping the exclusions resulted in a rate of 3.8/100 (Blazer, Hughes, George, Schwartz, & Boyer, 1991). Lifetime prevalence of generalized anxiety disorder in the ECA study was quite consistent across three study sites, varying from 4.1/100 in Los Angeles to 6.6/100 in Durham and St. Louis. In spite of differences in diagnostic criteria, the ECA and NCS rates of generalized anxiety disorder were quite similar. Lifetime prevalence varied considerably more in the Taiwan study, from 3.7/100 in Taipei to 10.5/100 in small town areas of Taiwan.

The Florence study provides an interesting example of the effects of requiring the longer 6-month duration of DSM-III-R. For DSM-III, the lifetime rate was 5.4/100, whereas the narrower DSM-III-R definition resulted in the lower rate of 3.9/100. In the NCS, which used a different interview (the UM-CIDI), the changes in criteria did not yield changes in prevalence.

Risk Factors

Based on data combined from three ECA study sites, the 1-year prevalence of generalized anxiety disorder, with or without diagnostic exclu-

TABLE 2.5. Prevalence Rates per 100 of Generalized Anxiety Disorder Using DSM-III (or DSM-III-R) Criteria

	Rate/100		
Place	6-month	1-year	Lifetime
United States: NCS (DSM-III-R)		3.1	5.1
United States: ECA (three sites)			
No exclusions		3.8	
No panic, no MDD		2.7	
United States: ECA (three sites)			
No panic, no MDD			
Durham, NC			6.6
St. Louis, MO			6.6
Los Angeles, CA			4.1
Zurich, Switzerland		5.2	
Florence, Italy			5.4
Florence, Italy (DSM-III-R)			3.9
Taiwan			
Urban			3.7
Small towns			10.5
Rural			7.8
Korea			3.6

Note. Adapted from Horwath and Weissman (1995). Copyright 1995 by Wiley-Liss. Adapted by permission.

sions, was significantly higher in females, in African Americans, and in persons under 30 years of age, but the differences were significant for age only without diagnostic exclusions and for race only when panic and depression were excluded (Blazer et al., 1991). The Taiwan study reported significantly higher rates for women than for men, but no gender differences were found in Korea.

OBSESSIVE–COMPULSIVE DISORDER

Definition

DSM-III obsessive–compulsive disorder requires the presence of obsessions or compulsions that are sources of significant distress or impairment and are not due to another mental disorder. Obsessions are defined as recurrent, persistent thoughts, images, or impulses that are experienced as senseless and repugnant. Compulsions are excessively repetitive, stereotyped behaviors, such as repeatedly checking locked doors or gas jets or washing hands (American Psychiatric Association, 1980).

Rates

Table 2.6 shows prevalence rates of obsessive–compulsive disorder from community studies using DSM-III criteria. Six-month prevalence of obsessive–compulsive disorder varied from 0.7/100 in Los Angeles to 2.1/100 in Piedmont, North Carolina. Lifetime prevalence of obsessive–compulsive disorder varied from 0.3/100 in rural Taiwan to 3.2/100 in Puerto Rico. The studies in English-language sites showed excellent agreement, with lifetime prevalence of 2.6/100 in the ECA and 3.0/100 in Edmonton, Canada. Most remarkable about these rates is that they contradict the previous traditional view of obsessive–compulsive disorder as a rare disorder, on the basis of published clinical reports.

Risk Factors

As with other anxiety disorders, prevalence rates of obsessive–compulsive disorder were higher among women than men in the ECA study. However, when gender comparisons were controlled for marital status, employment status, job status, ethnicity, and age, there were no remaining differences in prevalence rates for women compared to men (Karno, Golding, Sorenson, & Burnam, 1988).

ANXIETY DISORDERS AND DISABILITY ACROSS CULTURES

Epidemiological studies have shown an association between anxiety disorders and functional disability. Recently, the World Health Organization (WHO) Collaborative Study on Psychological Problems in General Health Care examined the relationship between common mental disorders and disability across cultures (Ormel et al., 1994). This WHO study collected data on psychiatric status and levels of occupational and physical impairment in primary care settings in 15 different sites around the world. Study sites included Ankara, Turkey; Athens, Greece; Bangalore, India; Berlin, Germany; Groningen, the Netherlands; Ibadan, Nigeria; Mainz, Germany; Manchester, England; Nagasaki, Japan; Paris, France; Rio de Janeiro, Brazil; Santiago, Chile; Seattle, Washington; Shanghai, China; and Verona, Italy. The investigators found that panic disorder and generalized anxiety disorder are strongly associated with functional disability and that this association is consistent across major cultures around the world. The consistency of the findings across cultures is of particular interest given the sub-

TABLE 2.6. Prevalence Rates per 100 of Obsessive–Compulsive Disorder Using DSM-III Criteria

Place	Rate/100		
	6-month	1-year	Lifetime
United States: ECA (five sites)			
New Haven, CT	1.4		
Baltimore, MD	2.0		
St. Louis, MO	1.3		
Piedmont, NC	2.1		
Los Angeles, CA	0.7		
Puerto Rico	1.8		
Edmonton, Canada	1.6		
United States: ECA (five sites)			2.6
Florence, Italy			0.7
Korea			2.1
Edmonton, Canada			3.2
Puerto Rico			3.2
Taiwan			
Urban			0.94
Small towns			0.54
Rural			0.30

Note. Adapted from Horwath and Weissman (1995). Copyright 1995 by Wiley-Liss. Adapted by permission.

stantial differences in cultural and socioeconomic environment across which this study was conducted.

CONCLUSIONS

In spite of the methodological limitations inherent to an epidemiological approach to cross-cultural research, lifetime prevalence rates of panic disorder are remarkably consistent across the community studies and across cultural, racial and ethnic boundaries, with the exception of the higher rates in the NCS, which may relate to differences in interview method, and much lower rates in Taiwan, where lower rates were reported for several disorders. Cross-nationally and cross-culturally, panic disorder is consistently associated with substantial levels of occupational impairment and is more common among women than men.

In contrast to panic disorder, the epidemiological data on agoraphobia show considerable variation in rates across studies and cross-culturally. A recent clinical reappraisal of the ECA data on agoraphobia without panic suggests that community studies relying on the DIS and DSM-III may have overestimated the prevalence of agoraphobia without panic. Therefore, the prevalence estimates from studies such as these should be regarded with caution until the accuracy of their prevalence figures on agoraphobia can be more thoroughly tested.

Analyses of relative risks showed higher rates of agoraphobia for women than men, just as with panic disorder. Unlike panic disorder, however, agoraphobia was associated with higher rates for African Americans than whites, and higher rates among those with less education or income. The differential effects of race and socioeconomic factors on panic disorder and agoraphobia suggest that the factors that cause panic disorder may not be the same as the factors that lead to the subsequent development of agoraphobia.

The ECA and NCS studies found that prevalence rates of social phobia were highest among women, those with less education or income, and those who never married. Generalized anxiety disorder was also more prevalent among women. Based on community data, obsessive–compulsive disorder turned out to be a much more prevalent disorder than suggested by previous clinical studies.

In conclusion, the cross-cultural data on anxiety disorders are interesting both for their consistency across quite different settings and for some of the questions they raise. Further study is needed to explore the consistently higher rates of anxiety disorders in women than in men, and to investigate the differential effects of socioeconomic and cultural factors on panic disorder and phobias. Increasing attention to the epidemiological study of anxiety disorders across cultures may contribute to our knowledge of the causes and treatments of anxiety disorders.

ACKNOWLEDGMENTS

This chapter was adapted from Horwath and Weissman (1995). Copyright 1995 by John Wiley & Sons, Inc. Adapted by permission. We wish to acknowledge the support of NIMH Grant No. MH 28274, "Genetic Studies of Depressive Disorders"; NIMH Grant No. MH 36197, "Children at High and Low Risk for Depression"; and an NARSAD Established Investigator Award, "The Continuity between Childhood and Adult Depression: A Longitudinal Study of Children as Depressed Adults."

REFERENCES

American Psychiatric Association. (1980). *Diagnostic and statistical manual of mental disorders* (3rd ed.). Washington, DC: Author.
American Psychiatric Association. (1987). *Diagnostic and statistical manual of mental disorders* (3rd ed., rev.). Washington, DC: Author.

American Psychiatric Association. (1994). *Diagnostic and statistical manual of mental disorders* (4th ed.). Washington, DC: Author.

Angst, J., & Dobler-Mikola, A. (1985). The Zurich study: V. Anxiety and phobia in young adults. *European Archives of Psychiatry and Neurological Sciences, 235,* 171–178.

Anthony, J. C., & Aboraya, A. (1992). The epidemiology of selected mental disorders in later life. In J. E. Birren, R. B. Sloane, & G. D. Cohen (Eds.), *Handbook of mental health and aging* (2nd ed.). San Diego: Academic Press.

Argyle, N., & Roth, M. (1986). The relationship of panic attacks to anxiety states and depression. In C. Shagass (Ed.), *Abstracts of the world congress of biological psychiatry.* New York: Elsevier.

Aronson, T. A., & Logue, C. M. (1987). On the longitudinal course of panic disorder. *Comprehensive Psychiatry, 28,* 344–355.

Barlow, D. H. (1988). *Anxiety and its disorders: The nature and treatment of anxiety and panic.* New York: Guilford Press.

Berkson, J. (1946). Limitations of the application of four fold table analysis to hospital data. *Biometrics Bulletin, 2,* 47–53.

Bland, R. C., Newman. S. C., & Orn, H. (Eds.). (1988). Epidemiology of psychiatric disorders in Edmonton. *Acta Psychiatrica Scandinavica, 77* (Suppl. 338), 7–16.

Blazer, D. G., Hughes, D., George, L. K., Swartz, M., & Boyer, R. (1991). Generalized anxiety disorder. In L. N. Robins & D. A. Regier (Eds.), *Psychiatric disorders in America: The Epidemiologic Catchment Area study.* New York: Free Press.

Breier, A., Charney, D. S., & Heninger, G. R. (1986). Agoraphobia with panic attacks: Development, diagnostic stability and course of illness. *Archives of General Psychiatry, 43,* 1029–1036.

Canino, G. J., Bird, H. R., Shrout, P. E., Rubio-Stipec, M., Bravo, M., Martinez, R., Sesman, M., & Guevara, L. M. (1987). The prevalence of specific psychiatric disorders in Puerto Rico. *Archives of General Psychiatry, 44,* 727–735.

DiNardo, P. A., O'Brien, G. T., Barlow, D. H., Waddell, M. T., & Blanchard, E. B. (1983). Reliability of DSM-III anxiety disorder categories using a new structured interview. *Archives of General Psychiatry, 40,* 1070–1074.

Eaton, W. W., Dryman, A., & Weissman, M. M. (1991). Panic and phobia. In L. N. Robins & D. A. Regier (Eds.), *Psychiatric disorders in America: The Epidemiologic Catchment Area study.* New York: Free Press.

Eaton, W. W., Kessler, R. C., Wittchen, H. U., & Magee, W. J. (1994). Panic and panic disorder in the United States. *American Journal of Psychiatry, 151,* 413–420.

Faravelli, C., Degl'Innocenti, B. G., & Giardinelli, L. (1989). Epidemiology of anxiety disorders in Florence. *Acta Psychiatrica Scandinavica, 79,* 308–312.

Garvey, M., & Tuason, V. (1984). The relationship of panic disorder to agoraphobia. *Comprehensive Psychiatry, 25,* 529–531.

Horwath, E., Johnson, J., & Hornig, C. D. (1993). Epidemiology of panic disorder in African-Americans. *American Journal of Psychiatry, 150,* 465–469.

Horwath, E., Lish, J., Johnson, J., Hornig, C. D., & Weissman, M. M. (1993). Agoraphobia without panic: Clinical re-appraisal of an epidemiologic finding. *American Journal of Psychiatry, 150,* 1496–1501.

Horwath, E., & Weissman, M. M. (1995). Epidemiology of depression and anxiety disorders. In M. Tsuang, M. Tohen, & G. E. Zahner (Eds.), *Textbook in psychiatric epidemiology.* New York: Wiley-Liss.

Hwu, H.-G., Yeh, E.-K., & Chang, L.-Y. (1989). Prevalence of psychiatric disorders in Taiwan defined by the Chinese Diagnostic Interview Schedule. *Acta Psychiatrica Scandinavica, 79,* 136–147.

Joyce, P. R., Bushnell, J. A., Oakley-Brown, M. A., Wells, J. E., & Hornblow, A. R. (1989). The epidemiology of panic symptomatology and agoraphobic avoidance. *Comprehensive Psychiatry, 30,* 303–312.

Karno, M., Hough, R. L., Burnam, M. A., Escobar, J. I., Timbers, D. M., Santan, F., & Boyd, J. H. (1987). Lifetime prevalence of specific psychiatric disorders among Mexican Americans and non-Hispanic whites in Los Angeles. *Archives of General Psychiatry, 44,* 695–701.

Karno, M., Golding, J. M., Sorenson, S. B., & Burnam, M. A. (1988). The epidemiology of obsessive–compulsive disorder in 5 U.S. communities. *Archives of General Psychiatry, 45,* 1094–1099.

Kessler, R. C., McGonagle, K. A., Zhao, S., Nelson, C. B., Hughes, M., Eshleman, S., Wittchen, H.-U., & Kendler, K. S. (1994). Lifetime and 12-month prevalence of DSM-III-R psychiatric disorders in the United States. Results from the National Comorbidity Study. *Archives of General Psychiatry, 51,* 8–19.

Keyl, P., & Eaton, W. W. (1990). Risk factors for the onset of panic attacks and panic disorder. *American Journal of Epidemiology, 131,* 301–311.

Klein, D. F. (1981). Anxiety re-conceptualized. In D. F. Klein & J. Rabkin (Eds.), *Anxiety: New research and changing concepts.* New York: Raven Press.

Kleiner, L., & Marshall, W. L. (1987). The role of interpersonal problems in the development of agoraphobia with panic attacks. *Journal of Anxiety Disorders, 1,* 313–323.

Lee, C.-K., Han, J.-H., & Choi, J.-O. (1987). The epidemiological study of mental disorders in Korea (IX): Alcoholism anxiety and depression. *Seoul Journal of Psychiatry, 12,* 183–191.

Lee, C. K., Kwak, Y. S., Yamamoto, J., Rhee, H., Kim, Y. S., Han, J. H., Choi, J. O., & Lee, Y. H. (1990a). Psychiatric epidemiology in Korea. Part I: Gender and age differences in Seoul. *Journal of Nervous and Mental Disease, 178,* 242–246.

Lee, C. K., Kwak, Y. S., Yamamoto, J., Rhee, H., Kim, Y. S., Han, J. H., Choi, J. O., & Lee, Y. H. (1990b). Psychiatric epidemiology in Korea. Part II: Urban and rural differences. *Journal of Nervous and Mental Disease, 178,* 247–252.

Magee, W. J., Eaton, W. W., Wittchen, H. U., McGonagle, K. A., & Kessler, R. C. (1996). Agoraphobia, simple phobia and social phobia in the National Comorbidity Survey. *Archives of General Psychiatry, 53,* 159–168.

Marks, I. M. (1987). *Fears, phobias and rituals.* New York: Oxford University Press.

Marks, I., & Lader, M. (1973). Anxiety states (anxiety neurosis): A review. *Journal of Nervous and Mental Disease, 156,* 3–18.

Noyes, R., Crowe, R. R., Harris, E. L., Hamra, B. J., McChesney, C. M., & Chaudry, D. R. (1986). Relationship between panic disorder and agoraphobia. *Archives of General Psychiatry, 43,* 227–232.

Ormel, J., VonKorff, M., Ustun, B., Pini, S., Korten, A., & Oldehinkel, T. (1994). *Journal of the American Medical Association, 272,* 1741–1748.

Pollard, C. A., Bronson, S. S., & Kenney, M. R. (1989). Prevalence of agoraphobia without panic in clinical settings. *American Journal of Psychiatry, 146,* 559.

Robins, L. N., Helzer, J. E., Croughan, J., & Ratcliff, K. S. (1981). National Institute of Mental Health Diagnostic Interview Schedule. *Archives of General Psychiatry, 38,* 381–389.

Schneier, F. R., Johnson, J., Hornig, C. D., Liebowitz, M. R., & Weissman, M. M. (1992). Social phobia: Comorbidity and morbidity in an epidemiological sample. *Archives of General Psychiatry, 49,* 282–288.

Thompson, A. H., Bland, R. C., & Orn, H. T. (1989). Relationship and chronology of depression, agoraphobia, and panic disorder in the general population. *Journal of Nervous and Mental Disease, 177,* 456–4633.

Thyer, B. A., & Himle, J. (1985). Temporal relationship between panic attack onset and phobic avoidance in agoraphobia. *Behaviour Research and Therapy, 23,* 607–608.

Thyer, B. A., Parrish, R. T., Curtis, G. C., Nesse, R. M., & Cameron, O. G. (1985). Ages of onset of DSM-III anxiety disorders. *Comprehensive Psychiatry, 26,* 113–122.

Torgersen, S. (1983). Genetic factors in anxiety disorders. *Archives of General Psychiatry, 40,* 1085–1089.

Uhde, T. W., Boulenger, J. P., Roy-Byrne, P. P., Geraci, M. F., Vittone, B. J., & Post, R. M. (1985). Longitudinal course of panic disorder. *Progress in Neuropsychopharmacology and Biological Psychiatry, 9,* 39–51.

Weissman, M. M. (1985). The epidemiology of anxiety disorders: Rates, risks, and familial patterns. In A. H. Tuma & J. D. Maser (Eds.), *Anxiety and the anxiety disorders.* Hillsdale, NJ: Erlbaum.

Weissman, M. M., Leaf, P. J., Tischler, G. L., Blazer, D. G., Karno, M., Bruce, M. L., & Florio, L. P. (1988). Affective disorders in five United States communities. *Psychological Medicine, 18,* 141–153.

Wittchen, H. U. (1986). Natural course and spontaneous remissions of untreated anxiety disorders: Results of the Munich Follow-up Study (MFS). In I. Hand & H. U. Wittchen (Eds.), *Panic and phobias* (Vol. 2). Berlin: Springer-Verlag.

3

An Overview of the Treatment of Anxiety Disorders: Focusing on Panic Disorder as a Model

LAWRENCE A. WELKOWITZ
JACK M. GORMAN

CLINICAL DESCRIPTION AND COMPARISON

Of all the primary anxiety disorders, including panic disorder, social phobia, specific phobia, obsessive–compulsive disorder, generalized anxiety disorder, and posttraumatic stress disorder, panic disorder is perhaps the most disabling in terms of interference with social and occupational functioning (Markowitz, Weissman, Ouellette, & Lieb, 1989). Panic disorder sufferers experience distress in the form of sudden, unexpected bursts of anxiety, which build to a peak within 10 minutes of their onset. This sudden ignition of autonomic arousal is accompanied by a minimum of four physiological and/or cognitive symptoms, including palpitations, shortness of breath, chest pain or pressure, dizziness or lightheadedness, hot or cold flashes, numbness or tingling, sweating, trembling or shaking, or feelings of depersonalization, as well as fears of going crazy or losing control, or fear of dying. Panic attacks often appear to occur in the absence of clear environmental triggers, as opposed to social-phobic reactions, which occur in social situations; specific phobia reactions, which occur in the presence of particular objects or events; or anxiety related to posttraumatic stress disorder, which occurs in response to recollections of traumatic events.

Although interview-based studies of the general population tend to show a high percentage of lifetime occurrence of a panic attack (from one to two thirds of surveyed populations), only a small percentage of these individuals develop diagnosed panic disorder. According to DSM-IV criteria, diagnosis of panic disorder requires recurrent panic attacks combined with a minimum of 1 month of either (1) persistent concern about having additional attacks; (2) worry about the personal, psychological, or physical consequences of an attack; or (3) a significant change in behavior related to the attacks. Panic disorder can occur either with a certain degree of escape- or avoidance-related behaviors (panic disorder with agoraphobia) or without agoraphobic avoidance (panic disorder without agoraphobia).

As with panic attacks, a high percentage of the population also reports some degree of distressing social anxiety. In one survey, Pollard and Henderson (1988) found an "unadjusted" prevalence rate of 22.6% exhibiting one of four specific types of social phobia, including public speaking, writing in front of others, eating in restaurants, or urinating in public toilets. The rate dropped to 2.0% when DSM criteria of significant distress were applied. Anxiety related to social cues is more predictable than that of panic attacks and diminishes reliably following removal of the feared social stimuli. Additionally, those with panic disorder, generalized anxiety disorder, or other phobias often feel comforted by the presence of others, whereas social phobic reactions are worsened by the presence of others. Social phobia may consist of isolated social fears, such as public-speaking fears, or may be more "generalized," thereby consisting of an array of social fears. Posttraumatic stress disorder and panic may often appear as one and the same, because posttraumatic stress disorder sufferers will often report panic attacks. Those suffering posttraumatic stress disorder, however, have experienced one or more traumatic events that are reexperienced in the form of distressing recollections, dreams, or dissociative flashback episodes. Additionally, those with posttraumatic stress disorder will exhibit persistent avoidance of events or stimuli related to the trauma, as well as symptoms of hyperarousal, including insomnia, irritability, difficulty concentrating, hypervigilance, and exaggerated startle response.

   Obsessive–compulsive disorder consists of either obsessions (highly irrational intrusive thoughts that persist despite attempts to ignore them) or compulsions (repetitive behaviors such as washing or checking) that are time consuming and interfere with daily functioning. Obsessive–compulsive disorder sufferers manage their anxiety differently than those with other anxiety disorders by engaging in typically "odd" ritual activities designed to produce short-term reductions in tension and discomfort.

EPIDEMIOLOGY

According to findings from the National Comorbidity Survey (NCS) (Kessler et al., 1994), lifetime prevalence rates for any anxiety disorder are 24.9% compared to 19.3% for any affective disorder. Although panic disorder may be the most commonly treated of the anxiety disorders, it is exceeded in lifetime prevalence by social phobia (13.3%), specific phobia (11.3%), and generalized anxiety disorder (5.1%). Separate findings from the Epidemiologic Catchment Area (ECA) program estimated a considerably lower lifetime prevalence for panic disorder of 1.57% (Eaton, Dryman, & Weissman, 1991). Data from the National Anxiety Disorders Screening Day (NADSD), which is based on a 1-day screening of over 16,000 individuals interested in seeking information and/or treatment for an anxiety problem, indicated a 1-month prevalence rate of 48% for panic disorder compared with 37% for social phobia, 17% for obsessive–compulsive disorder, and 14% for posttraumatic stress disorder (Streuning, Pittman, Welkowitz, & Guardino, 1996). Comorbidity was quite high, with panic disorder occurring alone in 5.3% of the cases, compared to 10.2% with panic disorder combined with generalized anxiety disorder, 7.9% with panic disorder combined with generalized anxiety disorder and social phobia, 3.4% with panic disorder, generalized anxiety disorder, social phobia, and posttraumatic stress disorder, and a surprisingly high 2.7% with all five major anxiety problems (panic disorder, generalized anxiety disorder, social phobia, obsessive–compulsive disorder, and posttraumatic stress disorder). High comorbidity rates found in the NADSD survey are consistent with similar findings from both the NCS and ECA studies.

   Panic disorder was found to be twice as common in women as in men. Lifetime prevalence rates of social phobia are also considerably higher for women, although men predominate those seeking treatment for social phobia. Age of onset for panic disorder is typically in late teenage years or early 20s, with onset in early adolescence or after 40 extremely uncommon. Obsessive–compulsive disorder is equally common in men and women.

PATHOPHYSIOLOGY

Family studies have suggested at least a moderate genetic influence on the development of panic disorder. Although obsessive–compulsive disorder is also believed to have a strong genetic component, there is a dearth of data on this and other anxiety disorders. The percentage of families of patients with diagnosed panic disorder with an affected relative are quite high (average equal to about 50%) compared to 20% for control families (Woodman & Crowe, 1995). Pauls, Noyes, and Crowe (1979) reported the rate of panic disorder in second-degree relatives to be twice that of the rate found in the general population.

Early twin studies by Slater and Shields (1969) and Torgersen (1983) found relatively high monozygotic (MZ) concordance rates versus dizygotic (DZ) rates among same-sex twins with "anxiety neurosis," an apparent forerunner of today's panic disorder. Several analyses of the twin data have yielded heritability rates ranging between 34 and 50% (Kendler, Neale, Kessler, Heath, & Eaves, 1993), thereby suggesting important roles for both environmental and genetic influences.

A major focus of pathophysiological theories has been abnormalities in respiration. Whereas a minority of panic patients have been found to be chronic hyperventilators, the primary abnormality is with the threshold for activation of the central carbon dioxide (CO_2) detection system. According to Klein's (1993) "suffocation false alarm" theory, the mechanism that signals suffocation, which is most easily activated in patients with panic disorder, is a rise in the concentration of CO_2. Psychological stressors may then act in concert with CO_2 hypersensitivity and the suffocation false alarm to produce panic attacks. Numerous studies have shown that patients with panic disorder are more likely to panic in response to biological challenges that create hyperventilation and hypocapnia, including injection of sodium lactate (e.g., Gorman et al., 1990) and inhalation of CO_2 (e.g, Gorman et al., 1994). This emphasis on respiratory factors, which underlies CO_2 hypersensitivity theory, has led to speculation that organic abnormality can be traced to respiratory control centers and noradrenergic and serotonergic nuclei and their connections with particular subcortical–limbic sites.

Recent biological studies of posttraumatic stress disorder suggest abnormalities in areas of the brain controlling memory function, thus

confirming findings of memory deficits indicated by comparatively
lower scores on the Wechsler Memory Scale (Bremner et al., 1995). Both
magnetic resonance imaging (MRI) and positron emission tomography
(PET) studies of posttraumatic stress disorder have shown both structural and metabolic differences in the hippocampus and amygdala,
leading to psychobiological theories tying traumatic stressors, changes
in neurotransmitter release, and permanent change in memory-related
brain structures. These alterations may explain posttraumatic stress
disorder sufferers' difficulties in retrieving particular memories, especially in the absence of trauma-relevant stimuli (Bremner et al., 1993).

ASSESSMENT

Reliable assessment of anxiety disorders is important, especially in
light of the high comorbidity of anxiety disorders and the importance
of understanding the details of the course of a particular patient's
course of illness. In our research programs, all patients undergo a
thorough psychiatric interview, followed by a complete DSM-IV Structured Clinical Interview (SCID) (Spitzer & Williams, 1996). Ongoing
information about course of treatment is collected via self-monitoring
of daily anxiety symptoms. Record-keeping methods are useful in
monitoring the symptoms of other anxiety disorders, including obsessive–compulsive disorder, generalized anxiety disorder, and social phobia. Weekly Clinical Global Impression (CGI) ratings by clinicians are
used to judge severity of the panic disorder and degree of improvement, both of panic symptoms and overall functioning, typically on
seven-point scales ranging from "markedly worse" to "markedly improved" (Liebowitz et al., 1988). Questionnaires that tap both cognitive
and behavioral aspects of panic and general anxiety, such as Marks's
Fear Questionnaire (Marks & Mathews, 1979) and the Hamilton Anxiety Scale (Hamilton, 1959), are more useful as outcome measures for
research compared to self-monitoring of symptoms and multidimensional ratings of improvement or impairment. For obsessive–compulsive disorder, patient self-monitoring of frequency and duration of
ritual behaviors provides desirable information for assessing severity
of illness as well as progress in treatment. Unfortunately, compliance
with such rigorous record-keeping methods is only fair to moderate,
necessitating the use of other assessment devices, such as the Yale–
Brown Obsessive–Compulsive Scale (Woody, Steketee, & Chambless,
1995) or the Liebowitz Social Anxiety Scale (Liebowitz, 1987). Scales for
posttraumatic stress disorder that have been rigorously validated are
not currently available.

TREATMENT

Nonpharmacological Approaches

There are two distinct approaches to treatment of panic disorder: a nonpharmacological cognitive-behavioral therapy (CBT) and treatment with medication. Although both approaches have shown a high degree of success, preliminary data from a large, multicenter study of panic disorder suggests that a combination of CBT and medication may be particularly effective. CBT often consists of 12 weekly 1-hour sessions focusing on management of both panic and generalized anxiety symptoms. The primary treatment components are (1) information on the nature of anxiety and panic, (2) breathing control and relaxation exercises, (3) cognitive therapy, and (4) exposure to interoceptive cues for panic (Barlow & Craske, 1989). The use of information about panic attacks is based on notions of the mitigating effects of stress inoculation (e.g., Rapee, Mattick, & Morrell, 1986). Breathing control exercises are designed to correct panic disorder patients' tendency to engage in rapid chest breathing, rather than slow diaphragmatic breathing. Cognitive challenge techniques are used to replace catastrophic thinking styles, which have a theorized connection to elevations in anxiety. Finally, exposure to interoceptive cues, by deliberately producing breathlessness via exercises such as breathing through a straw or dizziness by spinning in a chair, is based on a Pavlovian conditioning model that identifies subtle physiological events as conditioned elicitors of panic response. When panic disorder patients exhibit concomitant agoraphobic avoidance, behavior therapists will often supplement standard CBT with *in vivo* exposure to fear-eliciting situations, such as leaving the house or traveling on buses. Studies by behavioral researchers have shown success rates ranging from 80 to 90% (Barlow, Craske, Cerny, & Klosko, 1989; Craske, Brown, & Barlow, 1991). The efficacy of CBT has been corroborated by pharmacologically oriented clinicians (Welkowitz et al., 1991), although to a lesser degree. In our laboratory we offer patients participating in biological studies a choice between open treatment with CBT or medication and find a slight tendency for patients to choose CBT.

Other types of CBT have been shown to be effective in treatment of social phobia (Heimberg, 1989, 1991; Heimberg & Juster, 1994). CBT for social phobia consists of cognitive therapy designed to combat poor self-evaluations of social performance as well as in-session and *in vivo* exposure to feared social activities. The program developed by Heimberg and colleagues at the State University of New York at Albany (Heimberg, 1991) utilizes a group format that serves as the context for extensive role playing of anxiety-producing situations, such as dating, job interviews, or public speaking. Although a multicenter study comparing the monoamine oxidase inhibitor phenelzine and Heimberg's group CBT has not been completed, it appears that this behavioral treatment has both the high response rate and low relapse rate of Barlow's panic control therapy, and fares at least as well as medication treatment.

Behavioral therapy for obsessive–compulsive disorder is based on a "tension-reduction" model, which postulates an anxiety-reducing function of ritual (compulsive) behaviors. *Exposure* to anxiety-producing stimuli, such as germs or dirt for those with contamination fears, is combined with instructions to resist tension-reducing ritual behaviors (called *response prevention*), such as hand washing. Again, reported response rates are quite high, ranging from 80 to 90% (Welkowitz, Bond, & Anderson, 1989; Foa, Steketee, Grayson, Turner, & Latimer, 1984). Although there is clearly slippage across time, those patients who continue to practice exposure and response prevention techniques tend to maintain much of their treatment gain, and behavior therapy patients tend to show less slippage than patients treated with medication alone (O'Sullivan, Noshirvani, Marks, Monteiro, & Lelliot, 1991).

Few research studies have focused on CBT of generalized anxiety disorder or posttraumatic stress disorder. There is some evidence, however, that exposure based treatment of posttraumatic stress disorder may be helpful (Foa, Rothbaum, Riggs, & Murdock, 1991). A more controversial treatment that has received much attention recently is eye-movement desensitization retraining or EMD/R (Shapiro, 1989), a brief (two- to three-session) treatment combining induced eye movements with recall of traumatic events. Although the treatment is being promoted heavily by a group of behavioral research practitioners, others have rightly cited the need for rigorous outcome research. There is also limited evidence that combinations of cognitive and relaxation-based therapy is useful for treating generalized anxiety disorder (Barlow, Rapee, & Brown, 1992).

A common feature of all effective CBT approaches to anxiety disorders is *exposure* to anxiety-producing stimuli. Prolonged exposure directly affects anxiety by promoting acclimation to these anxiety-eliciting events or objects. The effects of exposure take place remarkably quickly, whether it involves a panicker's exposure to the symptoms of hyperventilation, the posttraumatic stress disordered war veteran's reaction to the sounds of a firefight, the social phobic's planned performance in a mock social event, or the obsessive–compulsive "washer's" deliberate exposure to sources of contamination. The success of this technique across the anxiety disorders suggests a psychological commonality among patients with anxiety disorders, namely, a persistent difficulty in tolerating discomfort in the form of anxiety symptoms. Exposure teaches anxiety patients that they can, in fact, tolerate greater amounts of discomfort than they had previously realized.

Medication

Selective Serotonin Reuptake Inhibitors

Our first-line medication treatment for panic disorder (as well as obsessive–compulsive disorder, social phobia, posttraumatic stress disorder, and premenstrual dysphoric disorder) is one of the four selective serotonin reuptake inhibitors (SSRIs) currently available in the United States: fluoxetine, sertraline, paroxetine, and fluvoxamine. Clomipramine is a tricyclic that also produces a specific inhibition of serotonin uptake in the synaptic cleft. Clomipramine was originally shown to be effective for use with obsessive–compulsive disorder, but has also proven to have antipanic effects (see Modigh, 1987). Three of the SSRIs have been approved by the FDA for obsessive–compulsive disorder (fluoxetine, paroxetine, and fluvoxamine) and three for depression (fluoxetine, paroxetine, and sertraline). Only paroxetine has been approved for the treatment of panic disorder. In one study (Oehrberg, Christiansen, & Behnke, 1995), the combination of paroxetine plus CBT resulted in a nearly 90% response rate for panic disorder. One meta-analysis of panic disorder treatment studies showed significantly larger effect sizes for SSRIs compared to benzodiazepines or tricyclics (Boyer, 1995). Another extensive meta-analysis showed larger effect sizes for CBT compared with SSRI, tricyclic, and benzodiazepine treatment, as well as lower financial costs for CBT (Gould, Otto, & Pollack, 1995). In addition to efficacy, all SSRIs have the advantage of minimal side effects and relatively low risk of lethal overdose. One way that SSRIs work to block panic may be by their direct effect on respiration, producing, for example, diminished sensitivity to carbon dioxide (Papp, Weiss, Greenberg, & Rifkin, 1995).

One negative effect of SSRIs is an "amphetamine-like" stimulation, which occurs in some patients during the initial few days of treatment. The intensity of this effect can be minimized by using a low dose, which can be increased following the initial 3–7 days of treatment. Full doses can be administered within 1–2 weeks of treatment. Effective antipanic dosages are 20–60 mg using fluoxetine or paroxetine, 50–200 mg for sertraline, and 100–300 mg for fluvoxamine.

The one controlled SSRI study for treatment of posttraumatic stress disorder (van der Kolk, Dreyfuss, Michaels, Shera, & Berkowitz,

1994) yielded fairly positive results using fluoxetine. Open trials using other SSRIs have also been promising, suggesting that this class of medications may be the first choice in pharmacological treatment of posttraumatic stress disorder.

Tricyclic Antidepressants

There is considerable evidence to support the efficacy of imipramine, as well as other heterocyclic antidepressants, in the treatment of panic disorder (Zitrin, Klein, Woerner, & Ross, 1983; Wilkinson, Balestrieri, Ruggeri, & Bleeantuono, 1991). Imipramine typically blocks panic within the first few weeks and is particularly effective in reducing agoraphobic avoidance. One problem is the moderately high side-effect profile, which includes dry mouth, hypotension, constipation, and weight gain. Nortriptyline is also an effective antipanic medication with somewhat fewer side effects and the added benefit of producing nighttime sedation for those whose anxiety is interfering with sleep. Nortriptyline produces antipanic effects optimally at a dose of 50–100 mg; the optimal dose of imipramine is 150–300 mg. Both imipramine and nortriptyline may produce initial amphetamine-like stimulation, which can be managed by administering low doses at first, as well as adjunctive use of benzodiazepines. Although tricyclic antidepressants may be useful for treatment of other anxiety disorders, they are no longer considered a first-line treatment. For example, imipramine and amitriptyline have been shown to be moderately effective for posttraumatic stress disorder (Davidson et al., 1990), but it remains unclear whether these medications are directly affecting core posttraumatic stress disorder symptomatology, as opposed to associated symptoms of depression and anxiety.

Benzodiazepines

Although alprazolam was the first medication approved by the FDA for panic disorder, problems of dependence and discontinuation have led clinicians to be conservative in its use. Alprazolam, along with clonazepam and lorazepam, are rapidly absorbed and rapidly produce antipanic effects, often within 1 week, with maximum benefits by 6 weeks. Although alprazolam may be administered in doses up to 10 mg, doses of 2–6 mg are most often sufficient (Uhlenhuth, Matuzas, Glass, & Easton, 1989). A requirement of higher than 6 mg may indicate increasing tolerance, which should elicit caution in planning further changes in medication dosing. The effective antipanic dose for lorazepam is 4–8 mg per day (Charney & Woods, 1989), and 2–6 mg per day for clonazepam (Raj & Sheehan, 1995). In addition to tolerance and dependence, other adverse effects of benzodiazepines include sedation (especially with clonazepam), intoxication, amnesia, psychomotor impairment, and a rebound of anxiety following discontinuation. It has been suggested that cognitive-behavioral techniques may be helpful in reducing this sudden return of anxiety while tapering benzodiazepines (Welkowitz et al., 1991).

Although benzodiazepines have not been well researched in other anxiety disorders, such as posttraumatic stress disorder or social phobia, limited information suggests that these types of medications alone are not effective in eliminating relevant symptoms, such as behavioral avoidance (Marshall, Stein, Liebowitz, & Yehuda, 1996).

Monoamine Oxidase Inhibitors

Although this class of medications was once branded ineffective for anxiety disorders, renewed interest in monoamine oxidase inhibitors (MAOIs) may be linked to Liebowitz's (Liebowitz et al., 1992) study demonstrating phenelzine's efficacy in treating social phobia. The Liebowitz study produced a 64% response rate at 8 weeks and a 76% rate for those with generalized subtype of social phobia at 16 weeks. Liebowitz and his colleagues used an initial dose of 15 mg, ultimately reaching an optimal dose of between 75 and 90 mg by the fourth week of treatment.

Despite its utility for both panic disorder and social phobia, practitioners are wary of prescribing MAOIs, such as phenelzine, because patients must adhere to a strict tyramine-free diet in order to avoid a hypertensive crisis, and because of the potential lethality in the case of overdose. MAOIs are obviously not recommended for patients with histories of drug and alcohol abuse or unwillingness to adhere to strict dietary guidelines.

Alternative Medication Choices

Controlled studies of the nonbenzodiazepine anxiolytic buspirone failed to fare well in comparisons with either alprazolam or imipramine (e.g., Sheehan, Raj, Sheehan, & Soto, 1990). Similarly, the antidepressant bupropion was shown to be ineffective for panic disorder (Sheehan, Davidson, Manschreck, & Van Wyck Fleet, 1983). Conversely, small to moderate success has been shown using clonidine (Liebowitz, Fyer, & McGrath, 1981), and the calcium channel blocker, verapamil (Goldstein, 1985). The most common combination of medications for panic disorder is that of an antidepressant, such as an SSRI, with a benzodiazepine. For social phobia, the most common combination is an SSRI with a beta-blocker. In the absence of sufficiently large clinical trials for social phobia, it is common practice to utilize beta-blockers for those with more discrete forms of social phobia, such as public speaking, and either SSRIs or possibly MAOIs for generalized social phobia. Benzodiazepines, such as alprazolam, and buspirone continue to be most often utilized for general anxiety disorder. While medication treatments for posttraumatic stress disorder await the development of further clinical trials, some novel pharmacological treatments appear promising, including the use of naltrexone for flashbacks (Bills & Kreisler, 1993).

TREATMENT RECOMMENDATIONS

There is little doubt that panic disorder, as well as the other primary anxiety disorders, will remain chronic conditions if left untreated. Although the symptoms of panic disorder may follow a pattern of repeated relapse followed by remission, other anxiety disorders, such as obsessive–compulsive disorder or social phobia, tend to maintain a level of symptomatology. The severity and intensity of posttraumatic stress disorder sometimes abate with the passing of years from the time of the initial trauma. The consequences of untreated panic disorder appear quite severe and include higher rates of cardiovascular disease (Kahn, Drusin, & Klein, 1987) and possibly higher rates of suicide.

In the absence of more information on the effectiveness of combinations of cognitive-behavioral and pharmacological treatments, we recommend that most patients with panic disorder, as well as social phobia or obsessive–compulsive disorder, consider a trial of behaviorally oriented therapy as outlined earlier. If symptoms either do not abate or become intolerable, medications are recommended as the next line of treatment. The advantages of beginning with CBT are (1) the patient learns skills for managing anxiety; (2) the patient tends to attribute success to his or her own efforts, rather than to the effects of medication; and (3) the patient may be less likely to relapse, particularly in the case of panic disorder or social phobia. Medication is particularly useful when the patient is having difficulty managing social and vocational activities, despite concerted efforts to overcome anxiety problems using only self-control procedures. Finally, there are some patients who prefer a medical approach to managing their anxiety problem either because of a personal view of anxiety as primarily a biological phenomena that is best treated with medicine, or because they are not interested in investing the time needed to practice cognitive-behavioral techniques in situations outside of the practitioner's office.

Although tremendous strides in the treatment of anxiety disorders have been made in the past 10 years, a number of important treatment issues have yet to be resolved. Perhaps most important is the question of whether behavioral and medication treatments lead to long-term alleviation of anxiety problems. Most follow-up studies have relied on greatly diminished samples of patients, making statistical analyses generally unreliable. Another important issue has to do with methods of assessing treatment outcome. For example, panic studies rely heavily on patient report of frequency of panic attacks during the past week. It may be that during CBT patients learn to describe panic attacks differently (i.e., learn new verbal behaviors regarding their panic attacks), leading them to conclude that physical sensations previously reported as full-blown panic are actually variants of generalized anxiety. This would result in artificially inflated estimates of recovery from panic for CBT patients compared with medication or control patients.

Finally, little is currently known about the demographics or cultural characteristics of anxiety disorder sufferers. For example, do older adults view anxiety symptoms differently compared with younger patients? Or, is there some biological explanation for diminishing incidence of these problems among older adults? Also, how do cultural factors affect the anxiety experience? For example, we know that in Japan researchers have identified a form of social phobia, which they call *taijin kyofusho*, in which the primary symptom is the fear of embarrassing others, rather than oneself. It is reasonable to expect that other variations of anxiety problems may exist that have been influenced by more "local" rather than universal social factors. Expanding the study of the assessment and treatment of anxiety disorders to more diverse populations may well lead us to new ways of conceptualizing one of the most widespread mental health problems.

REFERENCES

Barlow, D. H., & Craske, M. G. (1989). *Mastery of your anxiety and panic*. Albany, NY: Greywind.

Barlow, D. H., Craske, M. G., Cerny, J. A., & Klosko, J. S. (1989). Behavioral treatment of panic disorder. *Behavior Therapy, 20,* 261–282.

Barlow, D. H., Rapee, R., & Brown, T. A. (1992). Behavioral treatment of generalized anxiety disorder. *Behavior Therapy, 23,* 551–570.

Bills, L. J., & Kreisler, K. (1993). Treatment of flashbacks with naltrexone. *American Journal of Psychiatry, 150,* 1430.

Boyer, W. (1995). Serotonin uptake inhibitors are superior to imipramine and alprazolam in alleviating panic attacks: A meta-analysis. *International Clinical Psychopharmacology, 10,* 45–49.

Bremner, J. D., Randall, P., Scott, T. M., Bronen, R. A., Seibyl, J. P., Southwick, S. M., Delaney, R. C., McCarthy, G., & Charney, D. S. (1995). MRI-based measurement of hippocampal volume in combat-related posttraumatic stress disorder. *American Journal of Psychiatry, 152,* 973–981.

Bremner, J. D., Scott, T. M., Delaney, R. C., Southwick, S. M., Mason, J. W., Johnson, D. R., Innis, R. B., McCarthy, G., & Charney, D. S. (1993). Deficits in short-term memory in post-traumatic stress disorder. *American Journal of Psychiatry, 150,* 1015–1019.

Charney, D. S., & Woods, S. W. (1989). Benzodiazepine treatment of panic disorder: A comparison of alprazolam and lorazepam. *Journal of Clinical Psychiatry, 50,* 418–423.

Craske, M. G., Brown, T. A., & Barlow, D. H. (1991). Behavioral treatment of panic disorder: A two-year follow-up. *Behavior Therapy, 22,* 289–304.

Davidson, J., Kudler, H., Smith, R., Mahorney, S. L., Lipper, S., Hammett, E., Saunders, W. B., & Cavenar, J. O. (1990). Treatment of posttraumatic stress disorder with amitriptyline and placebo. *Archives of General Psychiatry, 47,* 259–266.

Eaton, W. W., Dryman, A., & Weissman, M. M. (1991). Panic and phobia. In L. Robins & D. A. Regier (Eds.), *Psychiatric disorders in America* (pp. 153–179). New York: Free Press.

Foa, E. B., Rothbaum, B., Riggs, D. S., & Murdock, T. B. (1991). Treatment of posttraumatic stress disorder in rape victims: A comparison between cognitive-behavioral procedures and counseling. *Journal of Consulting and Clinical Psychology, 59,* 719–723.

Foa, E. B., Steketee, G., Grayson, J. B., Turner, R. M., & Latimer, P. R. (1984). Deliberate exposure and blocking of obsessive-compulsive rituals: Immediate and long term effects. *Behavior Therapy, 15,* 450–472.

Goldstein, J. A. (1985). Calcium channel blockers in the treatment of panic disorder [Letter]. *Journal of Clinical Psychiatry, 46*(12), 546.

Gorman, J. M., Goetz, R. R., Dillon, D., Liebowitz, M. R., Fyer, A. J., Davies, S., & Klein, D. F. (1990). Sodium d-lactate infusion of panic disorder patients. *Neuropsychopharmacology, 3*(3), 181–189.

Gorman, J. M., Papp, L. A., Coplan, J. D., Klein, D. F., Martinez, J., Lennon, S., Goetz, R. R., & Ross, D. (1994). Anxiogenic effects of CO_2 with panic disorder and hyperventilation in panic patients. *American Journal of Psychiatry, 151,* 547–553.

Gould, R. A., Otto, M. W., & Pollack, M. H. (1995). A meta-analysis of treatment outcome for panic disorder. *Clinical Psychology Review, 15*(8), 819–844.

Hamilton, M. (1959). The assessment of anxiety states by rating. *British Journal of Medical Psychology, 32,* 50–55.

Heimberg, R., & Juster, H. (1994). Treatment of social phobia in cognitive-behavioral groups. *Journal of Clinical Psychiatry, 55*(6, Suppl.), 38–46.

Heimberg, R. G. (1991). *Cognitive-behavioral treatment of social phobia in a group setting: A treatment manual*. Albany, NY: Center for Stress and Anxiety Disorders.

Heimberg, R. G. (1995, July). *Cognitive-behavioral group treatment and phenelzine for social phobia: Posttreatment effectiveness and maintenance of gains*. Paper presented at the World Congress of Behavioural and Cognitive Therapies, Copenhagen, Denmark.

Kahn, J. F., Drusin, R. E., & Klein, D. F. (1987). Idiopathic cardiomyopathy and panic disorder: Clinical association in cardiac transplant candidates. *American Journal of Psychiatry, 144*, 1327–1330.

Kendler, K. S., Neale, M., Kessler, R., Heath, A., & Eaves, L. J. (1993). A population-based twin study of panic disorder in women. *Psychological Medicine, 23*, 397–406.

Kessler, R. C., McGonagle, K. A., Zhao, S., Nelson, C. B., Hughes, M., Eshleman, S., Wittchen, H., & Kendler, K. S. (1994). Lifetime and 12-month prevalence of DSM-III-R psychiatric disorders in the United States. *Archives of General Psychiatry, 51*, 8–19.

Klein, D. (1993). False suffocation alarms, spontaneous panics, and related conditions: An integrative hypothesis. *Archives of General Psychiatry, 50*, 306–317.

Liebowitz, M. (1987). Social phobia. *Modern Problems in Pharmacopsychiatry, 22*, 141–173.

Liebowitz, M. R., Fyer, A. J., & McGrath, P. (1981). Clonidine treatment of panic disorder. *Psychopharmacology Bulletin, 17*, 122–123.

Liebowitz, M. R., Gorman, J. M., Fyer, A. J., Campeas, R., Levin, A. P., Sandberg, D., Hollander, E., Papp, L., & Goetz, D. (1988). Pharmacotherapy of social phobia: An interim report of a placebo controlled comparison of phenelzine and atenolol. *Journal of Clinical Psychiatry, 49*, 252–257.

Liebowitz, M. R., Schneier, F., Campeas, R., Hollander, E., Hatterer, J., Fyer, A., Gorman, J., Papp, L., Davies, S., Gully, R., & Klein, D. F. (1992). Phenelzine vs. atenolol in social phobia: A placebo controlled comparison. *Archives of General Psychiatry, 49*, 290–300.

Markowitz, J., Weissman, M. M., Ouellette, R., & Lieb, R. (1989). Quality of life in panic disorder. *Archives of General Psychiatry, 46*, 984–992.

Marks, I., & Mathews, A. (1979). Brief standard self-rating for phobic patients. *Behaviour Research and Therapy, 17*(3), 263–267.

Marshall, R. D., Stein, D. J., Liebowitz, M. R., & Yehuda, R. (1996). A pharmacotherapy algorithm in the treatment of posttraumatic stress disorder. *Psychiatric Annals, 26*(4), 217–226.

Modigh, K. (1987). Antidepressant drugs in anxiety disorders. *Acta Psychiatrica Scandinavica, 76*(Suppl. 335), 57–71.

Oehrberg, S., Christiansen, P. E., & Behnke, K. (1995). Paroxetine in the treatment of panic disorder: A randomized, double-blind, placebo-controlled study. *British Journal of Psychiatry, 167*, 374–379.

O'Sullivan, G., Noshirvani, H., Marks, I., Monteiro, W., & Lelliot, P. (1991). Six-year follow-up after exposure and clomipramine therapy for obsessive–compulsive disorder. *Journal of Clinical Psychiatry, 52,* 150–155.

Papp, L. A., Weiss, J. R., Greenberg, H. E., & Rifkin, A. (1995). Sertraline for chronic pulmonary disease and comorbid anxiety and mood disorder. *American Journal of Psychiatry, 152,* 1531.

Pauls, D. L., Noyes, R., Jr., & Crowe, R. R. (1979). The prevalence in second degree relatives of patients with anxiety neurosis (panic disorder). *Journal of Affective Disorders, 1,* 279–285.

Pollard, C. A., & Henderson, J. G. (1988). Four types of social phobia in a community sample. *Journal of Nervous and Mental Disease, 176,* 440–445.

Raj, B. A., & Sheehan, D. V. (1995). Somatic treatment strategies in panic disorder. In G. M. Asnis & H. M. van Praag (Eds.), *Panic disorder: Clinical, biological and treatment aspects* (pp. 279–313). New York: Wiley.

Rapee, R., Mattick, R., & Murrell, E. (1986). Cognitive mediation in the affective component of spontaneous panic attacks. *Journal of Behavioural Therapy and Experimental Psychiatry, 17,* 245–273.

Shapiro, F. (1989). Efficacy of the eye movement desensitization procedure in the treatment of traumatic memories. *Journal of Traumatic Stress, 2,* 199–223.

Sheehan, D. V., Davidson, J., Manschreck, T. C., & Van Wyck Fleet, J. (1983). Lack of efficacy of a new antidepressant (bupropion) in the treatment of panic disorder with phobias. *Journal of Clinical Psychopharmacology, 31*(1), 28–31.

Sheehan, D. V., Raj, B. A., Sheehan, K. H., & Soto, S. (1990). Is buspirone effective for panic disorder? *Journal of Clinical Psychopharmacology, 10*(1), 3–11.

Slater, E., & Shields, J. (1969). Genetical aspects of anxiety. *British Journal of Psychiatry, 3,* 62–71.

Spitzer, R. L., & Williams, J. B. (1996). *The Structured Clinical Interview for DSM-IV (SCID IV).* New York: Biometrics Research, New York State Psychiatric Institute.

Streuning, E. L., Pittman, J., Welkowitz, L. A., & Guardino, M. (1996, May). *Characteristics of participants in the 1995 National Screening for Anxiety Disorders.* Symposium presented at the meeting of the American Psychiatric Association.

Torgersen, S. (1983). Genetic factors in anxiety disorders. *Archives of General Psychiatry, 40,* 1085–1089.

Uhlenhuth, E. H., Matuzas, W., Glass, R. M., & Easton, C. (1989). Response of panic disorder to fixed doses of alprazolam or imipramine. *Journal of Affective Disorders, 17,* 261–270.

van der Kolk, B. A., Dreyfuss, D., Michaels, M., Shera, D., & Berkowitz, R. (1994). Fluoxetine in posttraumatic stress disorder. *Journal of Clinical Psychiatry, 55,* 517–522.

Welkowitz, L. A., Bond, R., & Anderson, L. T. (1989). Social skills and initial response to behavior therapy for obsessive–compulsive disorder. *Phobia Research and Practice Journal, 2,* 67–86.

Welkowitz, L. A., Papp, L. A., Cloitre, M., Liebowitz, M. R., Martin, L. Y., & Gorman, J. M. (1991). Cognitive-behavior therapy for panic disorder delivered by psychopharmacologically oriented clinicians. *Journal of Nervous and Mental Disease, 179,* 473–477.

Wilkinson, G., Balestrieri, M., Ruggeri, M., & Bleeantuono, C. (1991). Meta-analysis of double-blind placebo-controlled trials with anti-depressants and benzodiazepines for patients with panic disorders. *Psychological Medicine, 21,* 991–998.

Woodman, C. L., & Crowe, R. R. (1995). The genetics of panic disorder. In G. M. Asnis & H. M. van Praag (Eds.), *Panic disorder: Clinical, biological and treatment aspects* (pp. 66–79). New York: Wiley.

Woody, S., Steketee, G., & Chambless, D. (1995). Reliability and validity of the Yale–Brown Obsessive–Compulsive Scale. *Behaviour Research and Therapy, 35*(5), 597–605.

Zitrin, C. M., Klein, D. F., Woerner, M. G., & Ross, D. C. (1983). Treatment of phobias I: Comparison of imipramine hydrochloride and placebo. *Archives of General Psychiatry, 40,* 125–138.

II

ISSUES IN THE TREATMENT OF SPECIFIC ETHNIC GROUPS IN THE UNITED STATES

4

Hispanic Americans

ESTER SALMÁN
KIMBERLY DIAMOND
CARLOS JUSINO
ARTURO SÁNCHEZ-LaCAY
MICHAEL R. LIEBOWITZ

The Hispanic population in the United States, now over 20 million and approaching 9% of the United States population, is growing rapidly. Since 1980, the Hispanic population has increased by 34%, compared to a 7% increase by non-Hispanics (AMA Council on Scientific Affairs, 1991; Malgady, 1994). In New York City, between 1960 and 1990, the Hispanic population grew from approximately 600,000 to 1.7 million, an increase of 290%; Hispanics now comprise 24% of the population of New York City and over 12% of the population of New York State (New York Magazine, 1991; Malgady, 1994). Given current trends, Hispanics are projected to represent the largest minority group in the United States by the year 2000. Although Hispanics in the United States share a common language, they are heterogeneous in terms of immigration history and national origins. Hispanic subgroups vary considerably in terms of the socioeconomic and demographic parameters.

In general, Hispanics are more likely than Anglos to be below the poverty level, without advanced education, underemployed, and without health insurance. Hispanics are at increased risk for medical conditions such as diabetes, hypertension, tuberculosis, HIV infection, alcoholism, cirrhosis, and specific cancers, and violent death (AMA Council on Scientific Affairs, 1991). Problems of language, culture, income, insurance status, and perceived health care needs work against effective utilization of health care services by Hispanics as a group in the United States. Additionally, it is important to mention that there are severe shortages of bilingual–bicultural Hispanic mental health providers in the United States. Surveying the major mental health provider organizations, the American Psychiatric Association in 1990 had 5.4% Hispanic members, the American Psychological Association, 1.6%, and the National Association of Social Workers, 2.6%. (Vargas & Willis, 1994). In New York City, where Hispanics comprise 24% of the population, only 5% (108 of 2,157) of the psychiatrists who are members of the New York County District Branch of the American Psychiatric Association are Hispanic.

DELIVERY OF CARE TO HISPANIC AMERICANS

For Hispanics, both language and cultural issues appear to contribute substantially to underutilization of the available mental health services (Rogler, Malgady, Costantino, & Blumenthal, 1987). Sue, Fujino, Hu, Takeuchi, and Zane (1991) found that Hispanics underutilized community mental health services. Collins, Dimsdale, and Wilkins (1992) found that Hispanics, as well as Asians, in the United States make less use of mental health services due to reliance on family support, religious beliefs, and traditional folk remedies. Poma (1983), however, found that the use of mental health facilities by Hispanics improved when bilingual–bicultural personnel were available, and stressed the importance of both language and cultural familiarity in servicing Hispanics.

The importance of the family in providing support to family members in a time of psychological distress should not be disregarded; however, it should also not be considered a primary cause of underutilization of mental health facilities among Hispanics. Hispanics living in the United States find themselves separated from their culture and their extended families, and therefore lack the support systems necessary to help their family members in times of crisis. Although Hispanic families have been typically viewed as close-knit and unified, conflict does exist, especially given the current increase in single-parent households. It has become more difficult for these families to help their relatives deal with mental health problems, thus increasing the need for help from professionals.

Additionally, cultural and language issues also pose barriers to obtaining effective medical or mental health treatment even after entering the health care system. Seijo, Gomez, and Freidenberg (1991) noted that Hispanic patients asked more questions and recalled more when seeing bilingual rather than non-Spanish-speaking internists. Hispanic patients are also accustomed to a paternalistic and medication-oriented approach on the part of physicians, including psychiatrists. Shapiro and Saltzer (1981) found an important effect of language similarity on the doctor–patient transaction, with better rapport, better explanation of the medical regimen, greater ability to elicit patient feedback, and greater patient understanding of the treatment when doctor and patient spoke the same language. Manson (1988) found that language-concordant care of Hispanic patients with asthma was better than language-discordant care.

In terms of mental health care, Sue et al. (1991) found that individuals who did not speak English as a primary language terminated prematurely and had poor outcomes in public mental health clinics unless they were both ethnically and language matched with the provider. Adams, Dworkin, and Rosenberg (1984) found that among patients at public mental health clinics in Los Angeles, Hispanics received less medication than Anglos and African Americans, and that this was a function of ethnicity as well as diagnosis. However, Flaskerud and Hu (1992) found no relationship of ethnicity to number of treatment sessions, treatment modality, treatment setting, and therapist's discipline in the Los Angeles county mental health system.

The few reports on treatment of Hispanics in the United States have also argued for the importance of language and cultural familiarity on the part of providers. Marcos and Cancro (1982) concluded that physicians treating Hispanic patients for depression must understand the psychological, sociocultural, and biological aspects of this population in order to develop a therapeutic relationship with the patient and to optimize pharmacotherapy. They suggest that the lower tolerance of Hispanic depressives to tricyclics is associated with the fact that Hispanic patients express depression in terms of somatic symptoms, which are often similar to the side effects of antidepressant medications. Thus side effects are often misinterpreted as a worsening of depression, leading to abandonment of treatment or noncompliance with the full dosage recommended. Ruíz and Ruíz (1983) also emphasize the usefulness of cultural and language familiarity in treating Hispanics for depression.

Unfortunately, bilingual–bicultural as well as just bilingual psychiatrists trained in the pharmacotherapy of anxiety and affective disorders are in very short supply and are not sufficiently available in many of the clinical settings to which predominantly Spanish-speaking Hispanic patients apply or are referred. In New York City, for example,

Hispanics comprise 24% of the population, but only about 5% of the psychiatrist population. As mentioned above, Hispanic psychiatrists comprised only 5.4% of the American Psychiatric Association national membership in a 1990 survey (Vargas & Willis, 1994). Accepting the fact that the treatment of Hispanics with poor command of English would be enhanced by knowledge of Spanish and familiarity with Hispanic culture on the part of those dispensing care, the question remains as to whether non-Spanish-speaking psychiatrists, if given some orientation to Hispanic cultural issues and utilizing bilingual–bicultural interpreters, can effectively deliver pharmacotherapy for conditions such as anxiety or affective disorders. Surprisingly, given the enormous need for psychiatric services among Hispanic Americans and the shortage of bilingual–bicultural and bilingual psychiatrists, the effectiveness of interpreter-assisted psychiatric treatment has not been prospectively assessed. In the absence of systematic data on trained interpreters, and based mainly on experience with untrained interpreters, standard practice at many clinical facilities entails placing monolingual Hispanic patients on substantial waiting lists or turning them away, and refusing to use interpreters, even though non-Spanish-speaking psychiatrists at those facilities are often less heavily utilized. These same facilities will use interpreters more liberally, however, to deliver non-psychiatric medical care to Hispanics. As a result, Hispanic Americans who are not English-dominant are being limited in their access to mental health services once the critical first step of seeking help has been taken. Often, Hispanic patients who do present for treatment are more severely ill in comparison to English-speaking patients with the same disorders—not because Hispanic Americans avoid seeking psychiatric treatment, as is often thought, but because their access to such services may have been restricted when their symptoms first emerged.

Thus, while effective communication with patients receiving pharmacotherapy is a prerequisite for safe and effective treatment, it may well be possible for non-Spanish-speaking psychiatrists trained to treat anxiety and affective disorders, and sufficiently familiar with Hispanic culture to achieve the necessary rapport and communication, to provide treatment, if trained bilingual–bicultural interpreters are used as well.

A number of investigators have documented the problems of trying to use interpreters to deliver mental health services to Hispanics, which include inaccurate summarization of what the patient is saying, intrusion of the views of the interpreter, and poor bonding between doctor and patient (Marcos, Urcuyo, Kesselman, & Alpert, 1973; Marcos, 1976; Marcos et al., 1979; Shapiro & Saltzer, 1981). However, these problems occurred when using family members, friends, or medical personnel without professional interpreter or mental health training. Acosta and Cristo (1981) found that, by using interpreters with language and medical training, briefing them before the patient was seen, and debriefing them after as well, mental health services could be delivered in a manner that greatly increased service utilization by Hispanic patients. Thus it may be possible that with proper training as interpreters, and with sufficient exposure to the mental health service environment, bilingual–bicultural interpreters could allow non-Spanish-speaking psychiatrists to deliver effective care to Hispanic patients. Prospective studies of interpreter-assisted psychiatric treatment need to be conducted in order to dispel possible misconceptions about this alternate system of treatment delivery, especially in light of the fact that large numbers of Hispanic Americans are not being well served by the existing mental health services.

VIEW OF MENTAL ILLNESS AND ANXIETY DISORDERS AMONG HISPANIC AMERICANS

As indicated, previous research has demonstrated that Hispanics underutilize mental health facilities. A variety of factors can explain why the Hispanic population tends to seek professional mental health care as a last resort. As mentioned earlier, the family acts as the primary caregiver for the mentally ill individual in the Hispanic community. In doing so, the family protects the patient from the embarrassment and vulnerability to criticism that is often associated with mental illness. The stigma of mental illness evokes shame and signifies a weakness in character. Therefore, the family often prefers to treat the illness as a "family problem" rather than a psychiatric illness. Studies of the cultural conceptions of the term *loco*, or crazy person, have revealed that this term is used to refer very specifically to psychotic-like symptoms—hallucinations and bizarre behaviors such as *hablando solo*, or talking to oneself. The stigma of being crazy not only evokes reluctance to go to psychiatric hospitals, but also evokes the suppression of psychiatric symptoms. "To be crazy is a sharply defined stigma and means losing all socially valued attributes. Crazy persons are seen to behave in ways that are antithetical to the society's value system" (Rogler, Malgady, & Rodriguez, 1989). In addition, Hispanic Americans tend to create culturally defined labels that they associate with mental illness, labels that often diminish help-seeking efforts. In our own clinic, patients often explain that they are seeking treatment for the anxiety or depression in order to prevent the illness from developing into craziness. These patients tend to view psychiatric symptoms on a continuum, and will fear, for example, that their panic attacks might lead to *locura* (craziness). According to Rogler et al. (1989), Hispanics delay treatment because they do not classify their symptoms as warranting professional attention until they become severe. Our patients often explain that prior to seeking treatment their relatives stressed to them that they had to *poner de su parte* or make an effort on their own to overcome their illness. Coming for treatment can therefore be seen as having failed themselves, or not having had enough strength to conquer the illness on their own. Their sense of shame and the value they place on pride serve as obstacles and contribute to the underutilization of mental health facilities.

In addition, the notion that psychiatrists are doctors that treat "crazy" people leads to further intimidation. The diagnostic labels given to the various psychiatric disorders accentuate the negative stigma associated with psychiatry. Gómez (1982) claims that, according to Hispanics, the diagnostic label stretches over the person: "Instead of being a functional description of a specific mental impairment, the diagnostic label serves as an ambiguous and pejorative statement about the patient's whole personality." For this reason, Hispanics often use cultural terms instead of the medical diagnosis when referring to the mental health problem of a family member. For them, these cultural terms signify a greater possibility for healing.

Guarnaccia, Parra, Deschamps, Milstein, and Argiles (1992) suggest that Hispanics view mental health on a continuum. At one end is the state of *estar nerviosa/o* (being nervous), which is due to situational distress. The next stage is *padecer de los nervios*, or suffering from nerves, caused by more enduring stress or perhaps the constitutional weakness of the patient him- or herself. The far end of the continuum Guarnaccia refers to as *fallo mental*, or mental failure. For Hispanics, this signifies craziness and little hope for recovery. Treatment should focus on getting the patient to the mild end of the continuum.

Acculturation also plays a role in how Hispanics view issues related to mental health. The higher the level of acculturation, the more likely it becomes that the Hispanic person will utilize mental health services. Rogler et al. (1989) confirms this finding and remarks that the lower the level of acculturation, the more likely it is for the individual to adhere to the traditional beliefs and perceptions of mental illness. They "are more likely than the acculturated to consider depression a more serious problem, they more often consider that mental illness is inherited, and more often view prayer as an effective mode of treatment."

Patients who enter the Hispanic Treatment Program at the New York State Psychiatric Institute tend to have a lower level of acculturation. Many of these patients live in Washington Heights, an area that is predominantly Hispanic (Dominican). Acculturation is not facilitated in this community as Spanish is spoken in the majority of businesses and public service offices, ethnic foods can be found in local stores or *bodegas,* and all close associates (neighbors, friends) speak Spanish as well. As a result, many of our patients still view mental illness in a more traditional manner, often associating mental illness with craziness. However, once our patients become educated about their illness (e.g., panic disorder), their new knowledge seems to take the shape of a "discovery" of sorts, and they feel compelled to educate others as well. For the National Panic Disorder Awareness Program, one of our Hispanic patients spoke on the radio (in Spanish) to relate her own experience, and we often find patients in our waiting room having an informal group session about their symptoms.

DIAGNOSTIC ISSUES AND
CULTURE-BOUND SYNDROMES

Of particular interest in working with Hispanic Americans and other "minority" groups is the realization that each culture colors and shapes its expressions of illness and disease. Some cross-cultural researchers follow the DSM framework, believing that these diagnostic categories can be validly applied to other cultures, provided, however, that precautions are taken to account for differences, for example in language, acculturation, and religious beliefs. In contrast, other researchers caution that such transpositions of diagnostic categories may not be valid; rather, such culture-bound expressions of illness should be studied independently, and these syndromes should not be assumed to be universal (Liebowitz, Salmán, Cárdenas, Jusino, & Davies, 1996). In response to the growing cultural diversity of the United States, the fourth edition of the *Diagnostic and Statistical Manual of Mental Disorders* (DSM-IV) has incorporated ethnically sensitive diagnostic formulations in the manual and accompanying sourcebook. Appendix I of DSM-IV (American Psychiatric Association, 1994) now includes a guideline for a cultural formulation that instructs clinicians to take into account an individual's ethnic and cultural identity before making a diagnosis; it also provides a listing of culture-bound syndromes.

Culture-bound syndromes have been defined as "recurrent, locality-specific patterns of aberrant behavior and experience which appear to fall outside conventional Western psychiatric categories" (Hughes, Simons, & Wintrob, 1992, cited in Parron, 1994, p. 21). This definition specifically refers to a pattern of behavior or actions that may not be captured by the existing diagnostic categories. However, this definition does not allow latitude for the understanding of otherwise diagnosable psychiatric disorders in non-Western populations, in a culturally specific and therefore relevant context. It could be proposed that the definition of culture-bound syndromes should be modified to a "recurrent, locality-specific labeling of a pattern of behavior or symptoms that may be generally captured by existing diagnostic criteria." How patients perceive and express their own distress is not only unique from culture to culture, but from individual to individual as well. In working with Hispanic Americans we have noted that what have been previously described as culture-bound syndromes within this culture may in fact be heterogeneous idioms of distress.

Ataques de Nervios

Ataque de nervios ("attack of nerves") is an illness category used frequently by Hispanic individuals to describe one or more particular symptom complexes. *Ataques de nervios* first appeared in the medical literature in 1955 with the work of Rubio and Doyle (1955), which focused on the extreme emotional reactions seen in Puerto Rican army recruits. Within a few years of its initial appearance, *ataques de nervios* came to be known as the "Puerto Rican Syndrome" (Fernández-Marina, 1959; Mehlman, 1961). Thus, *ataques* were regarded as a stress-related and culturally specific reaction. More recently, Guarnaccia, De La Cancela, and Carrillo (1989) have viewed *ataques* as a culturally shaped expression of emotion, which emerges specifically in times of severe stress.

Ataques de nervios usually occur at funerals, accidents, or family conflicts and will call forth family or other social supports, suggesting that they may be culturally shaped and sanctioned responses to severe stress (Guarnaccia, Rubio-Stipec, & Canino, 1989). Commonly experienced symptoms of *ataques* include shaking, palpitations, a sense of heat rising to the head, and numbness. The individual may shout, swear, and strike out at others; finally the person may fall to the ground and experience convulsive body movements—usually having no recollection of the event (Guarnaccia, De La Cancela, et al., 1989a). As such, *ataques* can be considered a normative reaction to stress.

Epidemiologically, studies have demonstrated that *ataques de nervios* coexist with psychiatric disorders. In a psychiatric epidemiological study conducted in Puerto Rico, Guarnaccia, Rubio-Stipec, et al. (1989) found that 23% of all subjects interviewed fit the category of *ataques de nervios* according to the symptoms they reported. A retrospective analysis of these data revealed that subjects with a positive history of *ataques de nervios* had elevated rates of psychiatric diagnoses. In a follow-up study, Guarnaccia, Canino, Rubio-Stipec, and Bravo (1993) found that 63% of subjects who reported an *ataque de nervios* met criteria for one or more psychiatric diagnoses, compared to 28% in those without a history of *ataques de nervios*. Thus, the findings of the initial report were confirmed, with *ataque* sufferers being 4.35 times more likely than those without an *ataque* history to have coexisting psychiatric conditions.

Clinical studies have also confirmed and extended these epidemiological findings. In a clinical study of 156 Hispanic subjects, Liebowitz et al. (1994) noted that 70% reported a history of *ataques de nervios*. *Ataques* were significantly more prevalent in females, with 80% reporting a history of *ataques* as compared to only 20% of the males. There was no difference in the prevalence rates between different Hispanic subgroups (e.g., Dominicans vs. Puerto Ricans). Additionally, individuals with and without *ataques* did not differ significantly in terms of current primary diagnoses, although *ataques* were frequently associated with one or more anxiety or affective disorders, including panic disorder, generalized anxiety disorder, recurrent major depression, and anxiety disorder not otherwise specified (NOS).

Of the 58 subjects who met criteria for panic disorder, 45 reported experiencing *ataques de nervios*. Of these subjects with both *ataques de nervios* and panic disorder, 80% seemed to be employing the term *"ataque de nervios"* as a self-label for their panic attacks. Additional analyses revealed that *ataque de nervios* was in fact a heterogeneous construct employed by Hispanic subjects, and that coexisting panic disorder, affective disorder, or other anxiety disorders correlated with distinct *ataque* symptom patterns. Those subjects with *ataque* and panic disorder reported the most asphyxia, fear of dying, and increased fear during their *ataques*. Subjects with *ataque* and an affective disorder reported the most anger, screaming, becoming aggressive and breaking things during their *ataques*. Those subjects with *ataque* and other anxiety disorders (i.e., generalized anxiety disorder, anxiety disorder NOS, social phobia, and obsessive–compulsive disorder) were not categorized by outstanding symptoms and overall exhibited less panic-like and less emotional/anger features during their *ataques* (Salmán et al., submitted for publication).

In summary, *ataque de nervios* in our clinical sample appears to be a folk label that is used to refer to several distinct patterns of loss of emotional control, some of which are diagnosable anxiety and affective disorders. It also appears that different subtypes of *ataques* exist, each subtype having a distinctive symptom pattern, and correlating with specific psychiatric comorbidity. Based on these findings, *ataque* symptoms may be a useful clinical marker for detecting the presence of psychiatric disorders. Clinically, it is important to understand the relationship between *ataques* and psychiatric comorbidity. Anxiety and affective disorders are highly treatable, and the danger is that Hispanic patients may be underdiagnosed for these conditions if they are being labeled as having only *ataques de nervios*, a condition for which no treatments have yet been proposed. However, further studies are needed to study (1) the temporal relationship of *ataques* with psychiatric disorders, and (2) individuals with *ataques* and no psychiatric comorbidity. Further validating studies, including biological studies such as CO_2 challenges could elucidate the overlap between *ataques* and panic disorder. In patients with panic disorder, 5% CO_2 will produce a panic attack in the laboratory, while producing no particular response in nonpanic cases. CO_2 challenges conducted with our patients who self-label what phenomenologically appear to be panic attacks as *ataques de nervios* could further validate that these "*ataques*" may in fact be panic attacks, if the patients have what they call an *ataque* and we diagnose as panic in response to the challenge. This result would further validate that there exists an overlap between the two phenomena.

Nervios

Nervios has been viewed as a "powerful idiom of distress used by Latinos to express concerns about physical symptoms, emotional states and changes in both the family and in broader society" (Guarnaccia & Farias, 1988). It is not a distinct loss of emotional control like *ataques*; it is more chronic and low-grade in comparison. *Nervios* are more transient than *ataques* and other mental illnesses. Hispanics often claim that their *nervios* "act up" at times and are provoked by external stressors. Whereas the Hispanic community views *nervios* as more of an emotional reaction, American families tend to view the symptoms as a medical problem (Guarnaccia, Parra, et al., 1992). Recently, studies have begun to assess the relationship between *nervios* and existing DSM categories.

According to Guarnaccia and his colleagues, untreated *nervios* can lead to DSM diagnoses. "There is a developmental sequence imbedded in these conceptualizations where untreated *nervios* can become mental disorders as the person's symptoms and behavior worsen" (Guarnaccia et al., 1992, p. 193). The Hispanic Treatment Program at the New York State Psychiatric Institute is currently examining the overlap of *nervios, ataques*, and DSM diagnoses. Although all of the findings are preliminary, the results thus far parallel the findings of Guarnaccia. Dominican and Puerto Rican patients are administered the EMIC, a culturally sensitive interview that surveys *ataques de nervios*. The goals of the interview are to reflect the patterns of distress, perceived causes, and general beliefs of people who suffer from *ataques de nervios*.

The initial data from the interview have produced interesting findings. *Ataque*-negative individuals seem at times to differ from *ataque*-positive subjects in their beliefs about their symptoms, rather than the actual symptoms experienced. That is, an *ataque*-negative individual may have *ataque*-like symptoms but not label them as such, saying that people who have *ataques* are more disturbed. After analyzing the responses of the pilot cases, the study personnel became more interested in the label of *nervios*. Hispanics make a clear distinction between someone who is suffering from *nervios* and someone who is "truly crazy." Patients feel more comfortable labeling themselves as having *nervios* because the condition does not imply psychotic symptoms. According to one patient, she has never had an *ataque de nervios* because she associates *ataques* with being crazy. People who have *ataques* "lose control, go into convulsions, start hitting themselves or the walls, and scream out of control at others. They are 'outside of themselves.' " She kept on repeating, "I am a sane person." Although she admitted to "slightly" suffering from *nervios*, the patient seemed hesitant to put herself in the same category as someone who has *ataquess de nervios*. She did not want to associate herself with the stigma that links *ataque de nervios* with *locura* (craziness), expressing the concept discussed earlier by which Hispanics view mental health on a continuum. However, the description of her *nervios* sounds like what another Hispanic would call an *ataque* and what an Anglo psychiatrist would call a panic attack: "I was watching TV and got scared all of a sudden. I started crying, felt dizzy, and had heart palpitations. I thought that I was having a heart attack." This patient prefers to use the cultural label of *nervios* to reduce the stigmatization associated with psychiatric illness.

The perceived causes of *nervios* also have captured the attention of researchers. Some Hispanics think that their weaker constitution makes them ill with *nervios*: "It's just the way I am," claims a woman about her condition, "every little thing makes me nervous." Other people talk of family conflicts or problems in their childhood that cause them to *suffer from nervios*. A patient interviewed in our *ataque de nervios* study thinks that problems with her children evoke her *ataques*: "They drive me crazy. Sometimes one of them will go out all night and I sit up worrying. My 19-year-old daughter fell in love with a married man. I got hysterical, lost all respect for her when I found out that she was no longer a virgin, and kicked her out of the house. I yelled bad things at her, like that she was not my daughter." After this episode, the patient went to see a psychiatrist and was given pills for *nervios* to calm her down.

A 31-year-old Puerto Rican woman participated in our *ataque de nervios* study after completing one of our social phobia protocols. The Structured Clinical Interview (SCID) showed that she met criteria for social phobia and subthreshold for panic disorder. Unlike most of our prestudy patients, who tended to be unsophisticated with respect to psychiatric terms, she differentiated between the panic attacks that she has when she has to give a speech in a classroom full of people and the *ataques de nervios* that she had as a little girl when her mother would hit her. She had her first *ataque* at age 6; she started to throw objects, scream, and break things. The patient describes herself as a shy and nervous child who was reared by strict parents. Her mother would never allow her to go out with other children and hit her a lot. She attributes the cause of her *ataques* to this oppressive family environment. These causes are consistent with the findings of previous research: "A stressful experience in one's childhood can leave a person's nerves permanently debilitated, putting one at a lifelong risk for developing nervous illness" (Guarnaccia et al., 1992, p. 194). Recently, studies have been interested in not only the overlap of *ataques de nervios* and DSM-IV diagnoses, but also the role of *nervios* in the patient's condition.

CULTURE-BOUND SYNDROMES:
THE NEXT STEP

At the Hispanic Treatment Program of the Anxiety Disorders Clinic at the New York State Psychiatric Institute, we have begun a study to assess temporal and phenomenological relationships of culture-bound syndromes such as *ataques de nervios* and *nervios* to existing DSM-IV diagnostic categories. Patients undergo a series of three separate interviews: (1) a structured diagnostic interview using the SCID to assess both current and lifetime psychiatric diagnosis; (2) a culturally sensitive interview using the EMIC, to elicit the patient's own view of his or her disorder in terms of *ataques de nervios, nervios,* or suffering from *nervios*; and finally, (3) a clinically integrative interview where the results of the two prior interviews are collapsed into a time-line that interweaves the patient's history in terms of psychiatric diagnosis and culturally relevant experiences. Table 4.1 outlines the initial results for the first six patients who completed all three phases of the study.

TABLE 4.1. Temporal Relationships of Psychiatric Illness and Culture-Bound Syndromes (*n* = 6)

Case No.	Sex/age/country	SCID diagnosis	EMIC diagnosis	Clinically integrative interview	Comments
1	F/61/Puerto Rican	Age 39: GAD Age 57: MDD	*Nervios* *Ataques de nervios*	Age 36: *Nervios*, could not sleep well. Age 39: First *ataque* following surgery. Age 39: Developed GAD following her *ataque*; became a severe worrier; further *ataques* in the face of big stressors such as family problems (4–5 *ataques* lifetime). Age 57: First MDD following severe family problem (grandson accused of rape).	Certain vulnerability (possibly behavioral inhibition) to anxiety and depression. Expressed in her idiom as *nervios* and *ataques*.
2	F/45/Puerto Rican	Age 17: SP Age 20: PTSD	*Nervios* *Ataques de nervios*	Unhappy, nervous, shy adolescent and child.	

(continued)

TABLE 4.1. *(cont.)*

Case No.	Sex/age/country	SCID diagnosis	EMIC diagnosis	Clinically integrative interview	Comments
3	F/26/Puerto Rican	Age 23: SP Age 25: MDD	*Nervios* *Ataques de nervios*	Age 10: Nervous as a child; trouble speaking up in school; she calls it *nervios*—nervous, jittery. Age 21: Started suffering from *nervios*—different from the *nervios* described at age 10. Life was stressful at this time. Had moved back to the United States from Puerto Rico. Age 23: Developed SP on her job; uncomfortable with coworkers. Did not talk to them, felt picked on and could not handle it. Age 25: Developed MDD—attributed this to difficulties with coworkers. Age 25: Started having *ataques* while traveling on the subway. Felt uncomfortable with other subway riders. Felt fine if she was on an empty car. Age 26: Quit job because of difficulties with coworkers, even though the supervisors liked her work.	Suffering from *nervios* indicated a more severe or pervasive condition when compared to *nervios*. *Ataques* experienced in the subway were not panic attacks—rather severe anxiety resulting from interaction with other people. Term "*ataques*" used to describe the SP.
4	F/35/Dominican	None	No *nervios* No *ataques de nervios*	No childhood history. Age 26: Beginning of intermittent depressive symptoms. Age 32: More persistent depressive symptoms.	

| 5 | F/31/Puerto Rican Age 18: SP | *Nervios* *Ataques de nervios* | Nervous since childhood, a very shy child. Had a very strict mother who would not allow her to go out with other children. Age 11–15: *Ataques* when her mother would hit her with a belt. Age 18: Developed SP, went to university, and could not talk in front of teacher or with a group. Age 21: Panic attacks after birth of son, intermittent panic attacks since then. Distinguishes between *ataques de nervios* and *ataques de pánico*. | Nervousness/shyness since childhood seems to be a marker for later problems. *Ataques* used to refer to episodes of loss of control—different than the panic attacks she experiences. |
| 6 | F/37/Dominican Age 37: MDD | *Ataques de nervios* | No childhood nervousness. Age 37: Six months prior to interview had onset of panic attacks; patient calls them *ataques de nervios*. Then developed anticipatory panic anxiety and agoraphobic avoidance. Age 37: Three months prior to interview had onset of MDD. | Self-labels panic attacks as *ataques*. |

Note. GAD, generalized anxiety disorder; MDD, major depressive disorder; SP, social phobia; PTSD, posttraumatic stress disorder.

ASSESSMENT AND TREATMENT OF ANXIETY DISORDERS IN HISPANIC AMERICANS

Help-Seeking Behaviors

The notion that Hispanics place a large amount of confidence in folk healing and spiritualists is a disputed theory amongst researchers. Although traditional healers, such as *espiritistas* (spiritual healers) and *yerberos* (herbal healers) may be sought for help with psychiatric symptoms in the countries of origin, in the United States reliance on these methods is somewhat less. Guarnaccia (1993) comments on the faith in religious beliefs held by Hispanics. God is seen as a doctor who will allow spiritual guidance to cure the patient. To some Hispanics, this faith in the spirits offers more consolation than the reassurance from doctors. However, we have found that among Hispanic Americans living in New York City, this scenario does not completely capture their help-seeking behaviors. Preliminary data from our ongoing study of *ataques de nervios,* in Dominicans and Puerto Ricans living in New York City have shown a different pattern of help-seeking behaviors. As part of the culturally sensitive interview, or EMIC, subjects are asked whether they sought help for their *ataques de nervios* from a list of resources including pharmacists, medical doctors, traditional healers, and so forth. Of the 28 subjects interviewed, only 1 had ever sought help from a *santero* (saint worker) or *espiritista*. The majority of the remaining 27 had sought help from either a psychologist or psychiatrist, a medical doctor or internist, or an emergency room.

Additionally, Hispanics who do seek treatment tend to identify themselves as "sick" and expect medication. Ramos-McKay, Comas-Díaz, and Rivera (1988) claim that Hispanics may get the medication, but may not understand how it should be used. They take it on an "as needed" basis and adhere to the general belief that too much medication is harmful. The Hispanic Treatment Program of the Anxiety Disorders Clinic at the New York State Psychiatric Institute has seen similar patterns. Patients often say that they have taken psychotropic medications "off and on" for a short period of time. We have seen patients who had been appropriately prescribed medications such as imipramine for panic disorder or fluoxetine for depression, but we found that these patients only took the medication when they had a panic attack or felt more depressed. Not surprisingly, they were disappointed when the medications had not worked as their doctors had promised. Others try to take less of their medication in order to save or conserve it because they think that they will not be able to get more. In our own experience, we have found that when patients travel back to their own countries they try to get the medication they need and bring it back to the United States, even asking relatives to do the same. Other patients anticipate a "miracle drug" that will work wonders overnight and lose confidence in the medication if it does not work right away.

Overall, patients seem to be poorly informed about how the medications work—how long it takes to see any change, how much and how frequently the medications should be taken, and what side effects should be expected. Patients have often come to the clinic with medication that had been prescribed previously in other clinics, and have not known why it was prescribed or what symptoms it was supposed to help them with. In our own research clinic, where lengthy, detailed consent forms are used for all treatment studies, we have found that too much information can also cause problems. Many patients become fearful of the medication when they read the consent that details all possible side effects; however, once each side effect is reviewed in terms of how frequently it usually occurs, the patients feel reassured. As with other, non-Hispanic patients we see in our clinic, the better patients are educated about their illness and the prescribed treatment, the better the rate of compliance. In general, mental health clinics need to implement psychoeducation in their programs; both patients and their families should be made aware of the various treatment possibilities.

DSM-IV Field Trial of Mixed Anxiety–Depression

The Hispanic Treatment Program participated as one of the seven sites for the DSM-IV field trial of mixed anxiety–depression. Our site was the only site that included Spanish-speaking subjects (n = 107); other sites that included both primary care and mental health clinics recruited predominantly non-Hispanic subjects. The field trial examined the prevalence of mixed anxiety–depression in patients that did not meet the full criteria for already existing anxiety and affective diagnostic categories. As compared to the other six sites, our site had the highest rates of coexisting anxiety and depression (19%) that did not meet full syndromal criteria. These patients would have been diagnosed as anxiety NOS or depression NOS. Interestingly, our anxiety NOS patients tended to report experiencing the somatic symptoms, but not the cognitive, worry features necessary to meet criteria for generalized anxiety disorder. Thus, it appears that the DSM-III-R did not provide adequate diagnostic coverage for Hispanic patients who were experiencing anxiety and depression sufficient to cause distress and impairment. The DSM-IV now includes a mixed anxiety–depression category in the appendix, which more accurately describes such patients with low-grade, but distressing and/or disabling anxiety and depression features.

Treatment of Panic Disorder with Imipramine

Patients with panic disorder were treated with imipramine after they either had failed to respond or were unable to tolerate a particular medication in a clinical trial. All of the 10 patients treated improved at least moderately over the course of treatment in a mean of 14 weeks (range = 8–26 weeks). The typical side effects seen with tricyclic treatment were reported, none of which interfered with treatment. The mean dose of imipramine was 102 mg per day (standard deviation = 29 mg), which is a relatively low dose; mean weight of the patients was 70 kg; and the dose/weight was 1.5 mg/kg. The blood levels were imipramine 74 ng/ml, desipramine 61 ng/ml, with a combined level of 135 ng/ml (Jusino et al., in preparation).

In comparison to previous studies, an open treatment trial by Aronson (1987) completed with Anglo subjects reported a mean dose of 130 mg/day. The blood levels were imipramine 62 ng/ml, desipramine 108 ng/ml, with a combined level of 170 ng/ml. In this study, a higher dose and higher blood level were necessary in order to produce a favorable response in Anglo patients.

A more recent study by Mavissakalian and Perel (1995), with Anglos as well, reported that the optimal plasma level was between 110 and 140 ng/ml. In this study, a dose of 1.5 mg/kg produced better results than a 3.0 mg/kg dose. With the 1.5 mg/kg dose (mean dose of imipramine was 99.1 mg per day, SD = 18.5) the blood levels were imipramine 42 ng/ml, desipramine 55 ng/ml, with a combined level of 97 ng/ml.

Recalling the study by Jusino et al., the dose of 1.5 mg/kg also produced the best dose range in Hispanic subjects. One notable difference, however, is that the Hispanic subjects had lower levels of the metabolite desipramine and higher levels of imipramine in comparison to the two aforementioned studies. If in a large sample this finding remains valid, it means that the Hispanic patients are not metabolizing the imipramine as quickly, and as a group there may exist some difference in the enzymes that produce the demethylation of the imipramine to desipramine. Clinically, this is significant because there may be more side effects for Hispanics associated with imipramine— the slower the individual metabolizes the imipramine, the higher the chance of experiencing side effects.

Previous studies of the pharmacokinetics of tricyclics have not shown significant differences in pharmacokinetics in Hispanics as compared to Anglos. In a retrospective chart review, Marcos and Cancro (1982) found that depressed Hispanic women received half the maximum tricyclic dose of Anglos, with comparable outcomes but more side effects. However, no blood levels were reported for this study. Gaviria, Gil, and Javaid (1986) noted no difference in the nortriptyline pharmacokinetics in Hispanic versus Anglo nondepressed volunteers. Mendoza, Smith, Poland, Lin, and Strickland (1991) also reviewed several of the enzymes related to tricyclic metabolism in Hispanics and Anglos and found no difference. To date, however, no study has reported on the enzyme that is specifically responsible for the demethylation of imipramine.

Treatment of Other Disorders

At the Hispanic Treatment Program of the Anxiety Disorders Clinic, other controlled clinical trials with panic disorder, social phobia, post-traumatic stress disorder, and hypochondriasis including clomipramine, moclobemide, fluoxetine, paroxetine, and imipramine have also not shown differences between Anglo and Hispanic patients. Although the details of these trials cannot be discussed at length here, there have been no differences between Anglo and Hispanics patients in terms of drop-out rates, response rates, tolerance to the medication, rate of success, side effect profiles, and placebo response. It can be concluded that, from a pharmacological point of view, the treatment of Hispanic patients with anxiety disorders, is quite similar to that of Anglo patients.

SUMMARY

In general, most Hispanic laypersons are not well informed about the current views of anxiety disorders or current therapeutic approaches. This is still seen to some degree in the Anglo community as well. Many of our Hispanic patients with panic attacks worry about having a medical condition despite medical evaluations that result in negative findings. Many fear that they are going crazy, believe that the disorder is their fault, and even worry that they are not trying hard enough to overcome their condition.

Anglo practitioners need to be better informed about folk diagnoses used in the Hispanic community as well as views of etiology. In our experience, it is reassuring to the patient when we conduct the EMIC, or culturally sensitive interview, and try to interrelate the patient's own experience and terminology (such as *nervios* or *ataque*) with the practitioner's formulation of the diagnosis. Using the patient's own term and showing the correspondence between the symptoms they describe and what we diagnose fosters a greater understanding of their illness and compliance with treatment. Thus, optimal care occurs when the practitioner's and patient's ideas on diagnosis, etiology and treatment can be reconciled. In general, practitioners need to be able to map the folk diagnoses onto the DSM-IV framework.

REFERENCES

Acosta, F. X., & Cristo, M. H. (1981). Development of a bilingual interpreter program: An alternative model for Spanish-speaking services. *Professional Psychology, 12,* 474–482.

American Psychiatric Association. (1994). *Diagnostic and statistical manual of mental disorders* (4th ed.). Washington, DC: Author.

Adams, G. L., Dworkin, R. J., & Rosenberg, S. D. (1984). Diagnosis and pharmacotherapy issues in the care of Hispanics in the public sector. *American Journal of Psychiatry, 141,* 970–974.

AMA Council on Scientific Affairs. (1991). Hispanic health in the United States. *Journal of the American Medical Association, 265,* 248–252.

Aronson, T. A. (1987). A naturalistic study of imipramine in panic disorder and agoraphobia. *American Journal of Psychiatry, 144,* 1014–1019.

Collins, D., Dimsdale, J. E., & Wilkins, D. (1992). Consultation/liaison psychiatry utilization patterns in different cultural groups. *Psychosomatic Medicine, 54,* 240–245.

Fernández-Marina, R. (1959). The Puerto Rican syndrome: Its dynamics and cultural determinants. *Psychiatry, 24,* 79–82.

Flaskerud, J. H., & Hu, L. (1992). Racial/ethnic identity and amount and type of psychiatric treatment. *American Journal of Psychiatry, 149,* 379–384.

Gaviria, M., Gil, A. A., & Javaid, J. I. (1986). Nortriptyline kinetics in Hispanic and Anglo subjects. *Journal of Clinical Psychopharmacology, 6,* 227–231.

Gómez, A. G. (1982). Puerto Rican Americans. In A. C. Gaw (Ed.), *Cross cultural psychiatry* (pp. 109–136). New York: John Wright PSG.

Guarnaccia, P. J. (1993). Ataques de nervios in Puerto Rico: Culture-bound syndrome or popular illness? *Medical Anthropology, 15,* 157–170.

Guarnaccia, P. J., Canino, G. J., Rubio-Stipec, M., & Bravo, M. (1993). The prevalence of ataques de nervios in the Puerto Rico disaster study: The role of culture in psychiatric epidemiology. *Journal of Nervous and Mental Disease, 13,* 275–295.

Guarnaccia, P. J., DeLaCancela, V., & Carrillo, E. (1989). The multiple meanings of ataques de nervios in the Latino community. *Medical Anthropology, 11,* 47–62.

Guarnaccia, P. J., & Farias, P. (1988). The social meanings of nervios: A case study of a Central American woman. *Social Science and Medicine, 26,* 1223–1231.

Guarnaccia, P. J., Parra, P., Deschamps, A., Milstein, G., & Argiles, N. (1992). Si Dios quiere: Hispanic families' experiences of caring for a seriously mentally ill family member. *Culture, Medicine, and Psychiatry, 16,* 187–215.

Guarnaccia, P. J., Rubio-Stipec, M., & Canino, G. J. (1989). Ataques de nervios in the Puerto Rican Diagnostic Interview Schedule: The impact of cultural categories on psychiatric epidemiology. *Culture, Medicine, and Psychiatry, 13,* 275–295.

Jusino, C. M., Salmán, E., Goetz, D., Arízaga, C., Vermes, D., & Liebowitz, M. R. *Treatment of Hispanics with panic disorder with or without agoraphobia with imipramine.* Manuscript in preparation.

Liebowitz, M. R., Salmán, E., Cárdenas, D., Jusino, C. M., & Davies, S. (1996). Nosological comments on culture and mood and anxiety disorders. In J. E. Mezzich, A. Kleinman, H. Fabrega, & D. L. Parron (Eds.), *Culture and psychiatric diagnosis: A DSM-IV perspective* (pp. 131–133). Washington, DC: American Psychiatric Press.

Liebowitz, M. R., Salmán, E., Jusino, C. M., Garfinkel, R., Street, L., Cárdenas, D. L., Silvestre, J., Fyer, A. J., Carrasco, J. L., Davies, S., Guarnaccia, P., & Klein, D. F. (1994). Ataque de nervios and panic disorder. *American Journal of Psychiatry, 151,* 871–875.

Malgady, R. G. (1994). Hispanic diversity and the need for culturally sensitive mental health services. In R. G. Malgady & O. Rodriguez (Eds.), *Theoretical and conceptual issues in Hispanic mental health.* Melbourne, FL: Krieger.

Manson, A. (1988). Language concordance as a determinant of patient compliance and emergency room use in patients with asthma. *Medical Care, 26,* 1119–1128.

Marcos, L. R. (1976). Bilinguals in psychotherapy: Language as an emotional barrier. *American Journal of Psychotherapy, 30,* 552–560.

Marcos, L. R. (1979). Effects of interpreters on the evaluation of psychopathology in non-English-speaking patients. *American Journal of Psychiatry, 136,* 171–174.

Marcos, L. R., & Cancro, R. (1982). Pharmacotherapy of Hispanic depressed patients: Clinical observations. *American Journal of Psychotherapy, 36,* 505–512.

Marcos, L. R., Urcuyo, L., Kesselman, M., & Alpert, M. (1973). The language barrier in evaluating Spanish-American patients. *Archives of General Psychiatry, 29,* 655–659.

Mavissakalian, M. R., & Perel, J. M. (1995). Imipramine treatment of panic disorder with agoraphobia: Dose ranging and plasma level–response relationships. *American Journal of Psychiatry, 152,* 673–682.

Mehlman, R. D. (1961). The Puerto Rican syndrome. *American Journal of Psychiatry, 118,* 328–332.

Mendoza, R., Smith, M. W., Poland, R. E., Lin, K.-M., & Strickland, T. L. (1991). Ethnic psychopharmacology: The Hispanic and native American perspective. *Psychopharmacology Bulletin, 27,* 449–461.

New York Magazine. (1991, June 10). p. 33.

Parron, D. L. (1994). DSM-IV: Making it culturally relevant. In S. Friedman (Ed.), *Anxiety disorders in African Americans* (pp. 15–25). New York: Springer.

Poma, P. A. (1983). Hispanic cultural influences on medical practice. *Journal of the National Medical Association, 75,* 941–946.

Ramos-McKay, J. M., Comas-Díaz, L., & Rivera, L. A. (1988). Puerto Ricans. In L. Comas-Díaz & E. E. H. Griffith (Eds.), *Clinical guidelines in cross-culture mental health* (pp. 204–232). New York: Wiley.

Rogler, L. H., Malgady, R. G., Costantino, G., & Blumenthal, R. (1987). What do culturally sensitive mental health services mean? The case of Hispanics. *American Psychologist, 42,* 565–570.

Rogler, L. H., Malgady, R. G., & Rodriguez, O. (1989). *Hispanics and mental health: A framework for research.* Malaba, FL: Krieger.

Rubio, M., Urdaneta, M., & Doyle, J. L. (1955). Psychopathological reaction patterns in the Antilles command. *U.S. Armed Forces Medical Journal, 6,* 1767–1772.

Ruíz, P., & Ruíz, P. P. (1983). Treatment compliance among Hispanics. *Journal of Operational Psychiatry, 14,* 112–114.

Salmán, E., Liebowitz, M. R., Jusino, C. M., Garfinkel, R., Street, L., Cárdenas, D. L., Silvestre, J., Fyer, A., Carrasco, J. L., Davies, S., Guarnaccia, P., & Klein, D. F. (1996). *Subtypes of ataques de nervios: The influence of coexisting psychiatric diagnosis.* Manuscript submitted for publication.

Seijo, R., Gomez, H., & Freidenberg, J. (1991). Language as a communication barrier in medical care for Hispanic patients. *Hispanic Journal of Behavioral Sciences, 13,* 363–376.

Shapiro, J., & Saltzer, E. (1981). Cross-cultural aspects of physician–patient communications patterns. *Urban Health, December,* 10–15.

Sue, S., Fujino, D. C., Hu, L., Takeuchi, D. T., & Zane, N. W. S. (1991). Community mental health services for ethnic minority groups: A test of the cultural responsiveness hypothesis. *Journal of Consulting and Clinical Psychology, 59,* 533–540.

Vargas, L. A., & Willis, D. J. (1994). New directions in the treatment and assessment of ethnic minority children and adolescents. *Journal of Clinical Child Psychology, 23,* 2–4.

5

Caribbean Americans

SHARON-ANN GOPAUL-McNICOL
JANET BRICE-BAKER

Although there is an immense body of literature on the topic of anxiety, considerably less literature exists on its cross-cultural manifestations. The fourth edition of the *Diagnostic and Statistical Manual of Mental Disorders* (DSM-IV; American Psychiatric Association, 1994) defines anxiety as apprehension, tension or uneasiness that stems from the anticipation of danger, which may be internal or external. Any cross-cultural study of such a class of disorders should be aimed at answering the following questions. Can a direct causal relationship be drawn between an individual's culture and his or her symptoms of anxiety, and if the relationship is not causal, is there some other way in which the culture influences the course, maintenance, and elimination of symptoms? The former question is difficult to answer as it has always been a formidable task in psychology to state with a high degree of certainty that one variable causes another. When an individual presents him- or herself for treatment, the therapist is confronted with many aspects of the latter question. For example, in what way have cultural norms influenced when a person decides to seek treatment? Or, what indigenous treatments exist for dealing with anxiety?

Over the past 20 years, there has been a proliferation of literature on the psychological functioning of African Americans, Latinos, and Asians. In the United States, Caribbean immigrants comprise a particular subgroup of the African American population, although little research has been reported on their psychological well-being (Gopaul-McNicol, 1993; New York City Department of Planning, 1985). Recently there has been an upsurge of interest in the psychological and social adjustment of immigrants from the English-speaking Caribbean. Two factors can account for this interest: (1) Caribbean immigrants in New York City comprise approximately 33% of the immigrant population (New York City Department of Planning, 1985), and (2) an increase of Caribbean referrals to psychiatric hospitals and mental health clinics (Gopaul-McNicol, 1993) has been noted within the past 10 years.

In this chapter we will attempt to address the following issues:

1. A brief examination of the psychopathological disorders among Caribbean Americans
2. The concept of mental illness and psychotherapy among Caribbean Americans
3. Risk factors in the development of anxiety disorders
4. Principles of assessment for Caribbean Americans
5. An overview of treatment techniques for Caribbean Americans

In psychiatric settings, anxiety has been reported as the most frequent complaint among children and adolescents (Kashani et al., 1987; Kashani & Orvaschel, 1988). However, an intriguing paradox between immigrant status and mental health has been noted; although immigrants tend to report a high number of symptoms of psychological distress, when prevalence of psychiatric disorders is examined, immigrants tend to show lower rates of mental health difficulties than their U.S.-born counterparts (Burnham, Hough, Karno, Escobar, & Telles, 1987). Burnham et al. attributed this to the fact that immigrants tend to respond differently on a written intake form than on the actual clinical interview. These apparently disparate findings thus raise concerns about the validity of Westernized diagnostic criteria for immigrants as a group. DSM-IV, like its predecessors, assumes that, across cultures and across populations, people manifest psychiatric distress similarly. However, evidence from cross-cultural studies of depression and other mental disorders suggests otherwise (Marsella, Kinzie, & Gordon, 1973; Tseng, Xu, Ebata, Hsu, & Cul, 1986).

Anxiety engendered by social situations seems to be a universal phenomenon, but the social incidents preceding the emotional states and the responses to those events are, to some extent, culture specific (Mesquite & Frida, 1992). An examination of the differences and similarities in the expression of anxiety in the Caribbean versus the United

States could shed some light on the conceptualization and boundaries of anxiety disorders among Caribbean people.

PSYCHOPATHOLOGICAL DISORDERS AMONG CARIBBEAN AMERICANS

Although many disorders are seen in many cultures, the manifestation and acceptance of these disorders depend on the cultural values (Draguns, 1987; Ponterotto, Casas, Suzuki, & Alexander, 1995). In the Caribbean, mood (e.g., depression) and anxiety disorders appear to be more prevalent and clearly are more acceptable to the patient and his or her family than personality and thought disorders (Gopaul-McNicol, 1993). In the Caribbean, repression of one's sexuality creates difficulties that are seen in a more psychosomatic manner such as vague physical aches, pains, dizziness, upset stomach, gas problems (mainly reported in the stomach), and nerves. These psychosomatic complaints often mask a depressive type of disorder that the individual, for cultural reasons, is unable to talk about it. Physical complaints are more accepted than psychological ones, and this may lead to difficulty in directly speaking about depression. Most people in the Caribbean have not conceptualized psychotherapy in the same manner as Westerners have, and physical complaints elicit much compassion from others, whereas psychological complaints result in a sense of weakness and failure, especially for men. Thus physical complaints often have secondary benefits because the person is relieved of his or her responsibilities because of these ailments. A classic example is captured in the vignette below:

> Mrs. P. was married for 8 years and had three children. Her husband left most of the family responsibility up to her, spending the majority of his free time with his mother and brothers. It is not unusual in the Trinidadian and Tobagonian society for men to put more emphasis on their family of origin, especially attending to their mothers over their wives. Mrs. P. was unable to change this situation by engaging in meaningful dialogue because her husband saw her as selfish and controlling when she requested that he stay at home more. Suddenly she developed many ailments, which were diagnosed as nerves. She was given Valium to address the "physical problem." This resulted in complaints of stomachaches, dizziness, and the inability to carry out the usual household chores. Mr. P. was forced to take a more active role in the home and to take her to and from the doctor. It was our impression that through these psychosomatic complaints Mrs. P. got

her spouse to spend more time at home and to be more involved in the domestic responsibilities.

CONCEPT OF MENTAL ILLNESS AND PSYCHOTHERAPY AMONG CARIBBEAN AMERICANS

In counseling Caribbean families, it is first necessary to examine two major cultural issues that may impact on treatment: (1) the concept of psychotherapy for Caribbeans, and (2) the therapeutic alliance.

The Concept of Psychotherapy

Due to a lack of exposure to and familiarity with the field of mental health in their home countries, Caribbeans generally do not readily accept psychological intervention. They tend to seek the help of a psychotherapist as a last resort. Another impediment to accepting psychotherapy is the social stigma attached to it. The average Caribbean believes that a person is either normal or "crazy," and only "crazy" people seek psychotherapeutic help. There is little perception of a continuum of behaviors between these two extreme points. In addition, few believe that intervention may prevent things from worsening. The therapist must be sensitive to these issues if therapy is to be successful. The therapist can assist the family by demystifying the concept of mental illness, while at the same time respecting this deep-seated cultural belief.

> The Matthews family was referred for therapy due to the academic and behavioral difficulties of their two children. At the very first session, Mrs. Matthews expressed concern that "my entire family will be seen as crazy because we are seeing you." This concern led to the parents being resistant to treatment, saying that they hoped the children would show improvement immediately, so they would not have to return for more than one session. In that first session, the therapist explained that psychologists see people with a variety of concerns, some of which may simply involve decisions on careers and so forth. Questions followed about the roles of psychologists and the types of cases the therapist normally sees. The therapist encouraged and responded to all of their questions, while simultaneously agreeing with the family that weekly sessions were indeed an inconvenience to all. Mr. Matthews was particularly pleased that "you [the therapist] understand and respect the fact that we do not really care for this." He nevertheless agreed to try treatment for 6 weeks, and

then evaluate if they wanted to continue for more sessions. By the time treatment had terminated, the family had stayed for 6 months and experienced much growth in all areas of concern that led to their referral.

The Therapeutic Alliance

In establishing a successful therapeutic alliance, one must begin by examining the client's expectations of the therapist and vice versa. Once a Caribbean patient and/or family have agreed to therapy, they tend to perceive the therapist as an expert—a problem solver who will guide the family in the right direction. The therapist, like a teacher or medical doctor, is seen as an authority figure to be respected.

However, if the therapist does not fulfill the expectations of the family, he or she will quickly lose their respect, and treatment will be terminated. In general, Caribbeans want a psychotherapist to be active and directive, yet personal, warm, empathetic, and respectful of the family's structure and boundaries. Being active and directive does not mean telling clients what to do or how to live their lives, nor does it mean being blunt and insensitive; rather it means taking initiative and directing the process of the session. For example, the therapist may give some direction as to which family member should speak first. It is recommended that, in keeping with the traditional family structure, the husband ought to be addressed first, then the wife, and then the children, according to their ages. If the wife is the one doing most of the talking, the therapist should attempt to assist the husband in commenting on her statements. If he is in agreement with his wife, the therapist can mention this to reinforce their unity; in some cases, the man's silence may be indicative of his strength and the respect he has for his wife's ability to understand the problems of their children. If he disagrees with her, the therapist can point out the validity of their different perspectives and attempts at different solutions, while attempting to address the disagreements.

Caribbeans, especially men, rarely initiate therapy because of marital problems. Those who do so tend to be more acculturated to American society. Most families who seek help in clinical settings do so because of a child's problem for which a medical doctor was unable to find a physiological cause. Hence, much of this chapter will address the needs of children and their families. The alliance with children in therapy often depends on their age. With adolescents, it is important to remember that they may have difficulty speaking in front of their parents, especially their fathers, particularly if topics to be discussed include drugs, sex, home conflicts, and school problems. It is important and beneficial to hear the adolescent's concerns in private. It is equally important to convince the parents of the importance of doing this. Caribbean parents will not automatically respect or even understand this need for confidentiality; for them, confidentiality is neither a right nor a given. But if they believe that part of solving the problem involves the acceptance of this process, they will be conciliatory to the therapist's request that they leave the room. However, some Caribbean parents will feel betrayed because, for the most part, they expect the therapist to support the parents' position. The goal of the therapy, of course, should be to help the adolescent to express his or her concerns to the parents directly and to find ways in which children and parents can forge a compromise.

In initiating and maintaining a relationship with a Caribbean client, it may be quite helpful to make a home visit. This personalizes the relationship and increases trust. In addition, a bit of self-disclosure (but not too much—always a difficult task for the therapist) is helpful in establishing a successful therapeutic alliance. This gives the family some perspective on the therapist. Obviously, this does not mean telling one's life story or becoming too casual; but if directly questioned, it may be helpful to reveal enough of oneself so the family sees the "human side" of the therapist.

It is important for the family to feel that they can disagree with the therapist. Because Caribbeans tend to confer a great deal of respect on a therapist once trust has been established, it is difficult for them to express anger or criticism toward the therapist, especially if the therapist has been helpful in resolving some family conflicts. The therapist must be responsive to nonverbal cues, such as changes in facial expression, sudden silence, or changes in vocal inflection, all of which may be indirect indicators that someone is angry or not in agreement with the current flow of treatment and is trying to suppress his or her feelings. Such suppression of feelings may also be noted among lower-status individuals toward higher-status individuals in the family. If not directly acknowledged and responded to, it is likely that this reluctance to open up may result in the family's abruptly terminating treatment.

In general, in order to establish a successful therapeutic alliance, it is necessary to explore the cultural strengths of the family; demonstrate a caring attitude; and be directive, warm, and "human," but not too friendly. In addition, it is best to be flexible with respect to home visits.

Resistance

In spite of all attempts to foster a therapeutic alliance, many Caribbean families remain resistant to therapy. Two factors in particular impact on resistance with the Caribbean family: the concept of time and family secrets.

The Concept of Time. Lack of observance of scheduled appoint-ment times is a major concern in therapy with Caribbean families, who often endorse the adages "any time is Caribbean time" and "better late than never." Culturally, Caribbeans tend to visit friends to socialize at any time without necessarily having received an invitation or calling ahead. Because of this informality, many clients miss appointments or appear at unscheduled times, expecting to be seen. It is important very early in the process for the therapist to explain the process of treatment. It is critical for the therapist to stress that timeliness is important because the family will have less therapy time for the same money if they come late. This will be quite effective, because, despite their tardiness, Caribbeans give priority to job demands. In fact, they often will not sacrifice their own work time for therapy, because they take very seriously the aphorism that "time is money." This behavior does not necessarily indicate "resistance" to therapy, but rather reflects financial demands on families with limited flexibility. A therapist may therefore have to be flexible in scheduling treatment so that therapy does not interfere with educational or work opportunities. If treatment results in the loss of money, the family or individual may, in fact, become resistant and resentful.

Family Secrets. Although Caribbeans may appear to be socially engaging, sharing "real family secrets" is a different issue. Secrets are to be kept within the family unit. Every child is told very early, "Do not put our business on the street." This means that openly and freely discussing personal and family issues with a stranger is often very difficult. Caribbeans also tend to deny family problems because they believe there is nothing that they cannot solve from within the family. They may often indulge in much circumlocution, especially in the initial stages of therapy. Thus, unless the therapist has clinical evidence that maintaining secrets is hindering the therapeutic process, the thera-pist is advised, particularly in the initial stages, to proceed on the assumption that keeping secrets may merely be a maneuver to keep boundaries in place. Pushing the family to tell their secrets too early in therapy may provoke mistrust and resistance, thus jeopardizing the therapist's position.

Perception of the Therapist by Caribbean Families

With Caribbean patients and families, once an individual has decided to go into treatment, the therapist is seen as an expert (Gopaul-McNicol, 1993). As such, the expert, or teacher, is supposed to solve the problem quickly. Thus, a short-term behavioral approach is more acceptable to Caribbean clients. In general, therapists are viewed as authority figures and are expected to play a significant and active role in the lives of their clients. A therapist is seen as powerful, a sort of scholar, but is still expected to respect the cultural boundaries while addressing the client's needs (Aponte, Young Rivers, & Wohl, 1995).

POSSIBLE RISK FACTORS FOR THE DEVELOPMENT OF ANXIETY DISORDERS

Immigration

Risk factors are those variables or situations that have the potential to make an individual or group of individuals vulnerable to developing a particular disorder. One potential source of stress for the Caribbean client is immigration. It is generally accepted that leaving one's country of origin and the circumstances around that event may result in traumatic reactions, with immigrants from Cuba and Haiti being good examples (Gopaul-McNicol, 1993). Large numbers of refugees fled from both these islands, mostly by boat and, to a lesser extent, by plane. Having to flee one's native country because of persecution, usually under life or death circumstances and often abruptly, with no chance to say good-bye to loved ones and no opportunity to plan or to bring one's belongings leads, naturally, to stress. The process may have involved living in constant fear of discovery. In addition, because of the secretive nature of these ventures, these trips may have involved boats or planes that were not sea- or airworthy. So even if one was able to escape, there was still the question of surviving the actual voyage. Those who did survive often are easily startled and experience post-traumatic stress disorder, with nightmares, flashbacks, hypervigilance, and difficulty concentrating. Often there is survivor guilt.

Another considerable source of stress for Caribbean immigrants, regardless of their reason for migration, is leaving family members behind. Sometimes anxiety symptoms are not even present until after the family is reunited. Having lived through separation in the past makes any future separation, real or imagined, a very toxic issue (Brice, 1982).

Once an individual or an entire family has successfully left the Caribbean, made connections in the United States, and established a home, other risk factors must be considered during evaluation and therapy. Adjustment disorder with anxious mood is a consideration when assessing reactions to a new home, a new physical environment, strange foods, and unfamiliar and brutal cold weather.

Dressler (1985) has posited another risk factor for stress associated with immigrant status. He suggests that being exposed to the American or Western lifestyle without adequate means to attain that lifestyle can make the Caribbean immigrant vulnerable for the development of symptoms. In his study, he tests the hypothesis that the greater the gap between the lifestyle the immigrant is exposed to and the immigrant's ability to attain that lifestyle, the higher the level of belief in witchcraft and the supernatural. His hypothesis was supported empirically in two of the three groups he examined.

Family therapists often get referrals when the family has been reunited. Such reunification calls into question family roles and family loyalty. Minuchin (1974) has stressed the importance of maintaining optimal family structure. Every family has a structure that provides family members with a blueprint for how to behave and knowledge of what is expected of them. It specifies gender roles (male and female) and generational roles (grandparents, parents, children). Minuchin and other structural family therapists (Kim, 1985) contend that alterations in the structure (i.e., boundaries between generations get blurred or members of one generation assume the duties of another generation) give rise to anxiety and symptoms in the family. The precipitator for the change in structure, the gradual or abrupt nature of the change, and the family's accommodation to it are just some of the factors that may influence who becomes the symptom carrier (i.e., the family member who develops a clinical anxiety disorder).

> Marie Chantal and her son, Jean Paul, left Haiti and traveled to the United States. Her husband, Jacques, was unable to leave the island with them; his parents were both ill and did not want to leave Haiti, and arrangements could not be made at the time for their care. When Marie Chantal arrived in New York City, she was quite overwhelmed. She began work as an au pair and was allowed to keep her son with her because he was only 7 years old. The biggest challenge for Marie Chantal was the language. She spoke Creole and very little English. Jean Paul spoke Creole but picked up English quickly as he played with the children of his mother's employer and started going to school. In time, Marie Chantal began to rely heavily on her son for translation. She took him to the immigration office, the bank, the market—almost everywhere she went. Jean Paul became a companion, of sorts, to his mother, but he also assumed a pseudoparental role with her. Several years passed and Marie Chantal found other work. She and Jean Paul moved into an apartment of their own. Jacques' parents died and he joined his family in the States. Much to Jacques' surprise and chagrin, his 11-year-old son was in charge of the house. Jean Paul spoke to his parents as if they were his equals. He helped his mother make major decisions and he didn't seem to take much stock of anything his father had to say. Not having had much recent contact with her husband and having had to rely heavily on her son, Marie Chantal was somewhat distant from her husband. Jacques'

frustration over his position as head of the family being usurped manifested itself in an "all-out campaign" to gain control. He became surly, often yelled about insignificant matters, and at times became physically abusive. As this went on, Jean Paul showed signs of increasing anxiety. The first visible sign was a drop in school grades due to difficulty concentrating on homework and tests. He was easily startled (in anticipation of his father's rages), had trouble falling asleep, was restless and irritable, and frequently complained of gastrointestinal distress.

This represents but one scenario in which anxiety and a full-blown Axis I disorder may develop in a family member because family structure has been altered and alliances of power have shifted.

Racism

Another risk factor is the experience of racism (Brice-Baker, 1994; Gopaul-McNicol, 1993). Racial discrimination is something that Caribbean and African American people share. However, there are some differences. Caribbean people of color have always been the racial majority in their countries of origin. They did not experience the lynchings, hosings, or Jim Crow laws that characterized the black experience in the United States. What both groups have experienced is a definition of who is black that has been imposed on them by whites (Gopaul-McNicol, 1993). In the Caribbean, considerable emphasis is placed on skin color because one's degree of brownness has been so inextricably linked to social class. It is shocking for the Caribbean immigrant on the lighter end of the color continuum to come to the United States and be relegated to the lowest rung of society. Anxiety can run high when an immigrant realizes that the lighter shade of his or her skin will not afford him or her any protection from discrimination.

Witchcraft

People from the Caribbean have not historically been major consumers of psychological services. Because of the diversity of ethnicities represented in the Caribbean, it is difficult in this short chapter to cover adequately the entire spectrum of indigenous sources of help. There are, however, some general statements that can be made regarding Caribbean attitudes about seeking help for emotional problems. Older people, particularly older family members, are thought to be imbued with wisdom. The opinions of men are given a great deal of weight, but there are certain areas in which women are thought to be better informed. Religion has also been a preferred method of coping with psychological problems (Brice, 1982). Catholicism is largely practiced in the Spanish- and French-speaking countries, whereas Protestantism is found in the English-speaking lands. *Obeah,* voodoo, *espiritismo,* and *santeriá,* among others, provide an adjunctive source of spiritual guidance to the above mentioned Western belief systems.

These non-Western belief systems are often referred to as witchcraft but such terminology could be considered a misnomer. In European countries, witchcraft has always been associated with anti-Christian and pro-Satan ideology, which obviously gives it a negative connotation. In the Caribbean, witchcraft does not involve devil worship. People consult the practitioners for many of the same reasons people seek psychotherapy. In his book *Working the Spirit,* Murphy (1994) quotes Edward Long, a historian, who summarizes the role of witchcraft (in this case, *Obeah*) in at least one Caribbean society (Jamaica):

> The Negroes in general, whether Africans or Creoles, revere, consult, and abhor them; to these oracles they resort, and with the most implicit faith, upon all occasions, whether for the cure of disorders, the obtaining of revenge for injuries or insults, the conciliating of favor, the discovery and punishment of the thief or adulterer, and the prediction of the future. (Williams, 1932, p. 113)

In a reference to the practice of voodoo in Haiti, Murphy (1994) states: "Oungans and manbos are also experts at feuilliages, the herbalist arts of physical and psychic medicines" (p. 19).

There are a couple of ways in which anxiety disorders and witchcraft may intersect. On the one hand, people suffering from anxiety symptoms may seek the help of witchcraft practitioners in order to obtain relief. On the other hand, an individual's fear of evil spirits or fear of being the object of an evil spell could possibly precipitate panic attacks. Sometimes elaborate rituals (almost resembling obsessive–compulsive disorder) have been developed by individuals desiring to ward off the evil spirits. Clinicians from outside the Caribbean may often overdiagnose psychopathology (i.e., psychotic disorder) when faced with culturally accepted behaviors and beliefs with which they are unfamiliar.

PRINCIPLES OF ASSESSMENT

There are several things that need to be included in an assessment of anxiety disorders in Caribbean people. To begin with, there are some overarching general considerations. Treating clinicians should try to avoid using a formal, stylistic mental status examination, in cases where one has been implemented, they should review the results with caution (Paniagua, 1994). Typically, certain questions used to test memory and intellect refer to knowledge about the United States, and its government, geography, and so forth. The assumption being that the average person living here should be able to respond to these questions. However, that would obviously not be the case with members of some minority groups and immigrants.

Responses to questions used to assess orientation may be vague or may come after a pause during which the individual searches for the correct answers. There are a number of cultures where little to no emphasis is placed on knowing the time or being on time. As previously discussed, the Caribbean is a place where time is fluid.

Another aspect of the mental status examination is an assessment of the individual's thought process, determining whether it is clear, coherent, and relevant to the discussion at hand. Circumstantiality, a common feature of obsessive–compulsive disorder, may be erroneously applied to clients from the Caribbean. Many of the cultures in this part of the world rely heavily on verbal as opposed to written communication. The telling of stories is one of the primary methods of conveying a point. Some of the better storytellers are revered community members, elders, and teachers. It is important to note that directness and getting to the point quickly are not desirable features in this age-old tradition.

Assessment of the level of acculturation is a critical aspect of the assessment process. Like a still painter's canvas, it provides a necessary background for the artist to shape perspective and eventually position the elements of what he or she sees. Although the therapist is not an artist per se, he or she must put the various elements of an evaluation into a framework that is as appropriate and accurate as possible. In order to understand what anxiety means to the Caribbean client, one should have a sense of the degree to which new cultural patterns have been integrated into the original cultural patterns (Dana, 1993). There are a number of formal acculturation scales already in existence for use with a variety of groups: the Behavioral Acculturation Scale for use with Cubans (Szapocznik, Scopetta, Arnalde, & Kurtines, 1978), the Cuban Behavioral Identity Questionnaire (Garcia & Lega, 1979), and the Brief Acculturation Scale (Burnham et al., 1987).

As part of the assessment phase, a clinician needs to be familiar with culture-bound syndromes. These are culturally specific disorders defined by the mores and belief systems indigenous to the Caribbean. The following brief list of disorders is germane to segments of the Caribbean population:

Ataque de nervios: out-of-consciousness state resulting from evil spirits (covered in detail by Guarnaccia, Chapter 1, and Salmán et al., Chapter 4, in this volume)

Falling out: seizure-like symptoms resulting from traumatic events

Mal puesto: hex, rootwork, voodoo death; refers to unnatural diseases and death resulting from the power of people who use evil spirits

Susto, espanto, or *miedo*: tiredness and weakness resulting from frightening and startling experiences (Paniagua, 1994, p. 113)

OVERVIEW OF TREATMENT

Indigenous Treatments

The treatment of anxiety disorders in the Caribbean is approached in a variety of ways. Consultation with a powerful witch doctor or spiritist is one method. These experts may offer help in the form of (1) medicine (herbal preparation); (2) insight into the spiritual forces, both seen and unseen, that may be at the root of the individual's anxiety; or (3) working spells on the person or persons viewed as the source of stress. Dressler (1985) suggests a fourth, almost psychodynamic, role for witchcraft in the alleviation of stress and anxiety: "These belief systems represent a culturally constituted defense mechanism because they enable the individual to resolve psychological distress, either arising from unconscious conflicts or social stressors, by displacing or projecting that distress onto beings inhabiting the supernatural world" (p. 275).

Another treatment method that has demonstrated substantial relief is Spiritual Baptist Mourning (Griffith, Mahy, & Young, 1986). This ritual is characterized by a 7-day period of isolation during which the individual prays, fasts, and experiences dreams and visions (Griffith et al., 1986, p. 226). In the Griffith et al. study, the Symptom Checklist 90—Revised was administered to the subjects pre- and postritual. Results indicated that there was no significant difference on the somatization dimension. However, the group reported fewer obsessive–compulsive symptoms and less interpersonal sensitivity, depression, anxiety, hostility, phobic anxiety, paranoid ideation, and psychoticism (p. 228). It should be noted that a major weakness of the study was the very small sample size, which severely limited the generalizability of the results.

Traditional Western Treatment

In this section we will briefly review some of the major DSM-IV diagnoses and some guidelines for treatment.

Posttraumatic Stress Disorder

General rules of thumb for treating Caribbean patients suffering from posttraumatic stress disorder involve prompt detection and treatment. The acknowledgment of immigration as a form of trauma and normalizing a person's reaction to the immigration process is often critically useful to the client and his or her family. The most significant difference between the Caribbean and the European immigrants' experience is the former's inability to blend into American society (no matter how acculturated, a person of color will always stand out) and their experience of racial discrimination. Attempts on the part of the therapist to draw parallels between the two experiences may be perceived by the Caribbean patient as a trivialization of his or her concerns.

Groups, of the therapeutic and support variety, are useful. It is important that Caribbean patients with posttraumatic stress disorder as a result of immigration not be placed in groups with other patients who are coping with a different type of posttraumatic stress disorder. There is too much of a risk for the scapegoating of this individual. The ideal situation is to have a group for recent immigrants focusing on a number of issues such as the reason for leaving, how the decision to leave was made, the burden of secrecy, the apprehension associated with survival, ambivalence about leaving family members behind, survivor guilt for having made it out and fear of possible repercussions for family members still at home. Another group can be geared for those individuals with a delayed onset of symptoms. The symptom picture is often the same for both groups with one exception; the delayed onset group may be at a different level of acculturation. They may also experience a degree of embarrassment that what they thought they had put behind them has come back to haunt them.

Obsessive–Compulsive Disorder

The first step in the treatment of obsessive–compulsive disorder is accurate diagnosis. It is important to determine whether or not the reported ritualistic behavior is culturally syntonic. If the behavior is not culturally prescribed and is interfering with the individual's social and occupational functioning, then intervention is called for. To the best of our knowledge, there are no controlled outcome studies but our impression is that a cognitive-behavioral approach may not be very effective for Caribbean clients because they often desire a more active approach. Reinforcement schedules that emphasize positive reinforcement for the absence of ritualistic behavior are recommended (Gopaul-McNicol, 1995). Also, this is a situation in which

Caribbean patients may be receptive to the prescription of psychotropic medication.

Generalized Anxiety Disorder

One of the keys to the treatment of generalized anxiety disorders in this population is removing the stigma of mental illness. It is important for Caribbean patients to hear the therapist say that what they are experiencing does not mean that they are crazy. This is a critical aspect in the psychoeducational phase of treatment (Gopaul-McNicol, 1995). It is also important for the therapist to provide some instillation of hope, by giving patients assurances that their problems can be dealt with. Too often Caribbean people think of mental illness, or "craziness," as static and unchangeable.

It is useful to get patients actively involved in their treatment so they can have the experience of efficacy. They can provide the therapist with a list of the conditions under which anxiety is experienced. They can rate the severity of their reactions. Family members can be included, helping the therapist to test the reliability of the patient's report. Seeing the entire family can also help the therapist decide if there is any secondary gain for the patient in continuing to present with these symptoms. The value of focusing on strengths and inherent coping styles cannot be stressed enough (Gopaul-McNicol, 1995). Many members of the Caribbean population are accustomed to being viewed from a deficit model, and a negative approach only reifies existing behaviors and drives patients away.

Panic Disorder

Once a differential diagnosis has been conducted, treatment of panic disorder with or without agoraphobia involves blocking of the panic attacks and brief psychotherapy (Barlow & Cerny, 1988). Reassuring the patient that the symptoms can be managed and are often transient is necessary for panic disorder with or without agoraphobia. Some psychotropic drugs such as benzodiazepines or antidepressants (although not necessarily viewed in the same manner as depression) are more commonly accepted than antipsychotics and utilized by Caribbean families. Although these drugs may aid in mitigating anticipatory anxiety, Caribbean patients tend to respond more to reassurances from the therapist that they can control their anxiety with behavioral interventions. Thus, Caribbean patients as a whole do not appear to require medication for long periods of time. Effective behavioral interventions include *in vivo* desensitization, exposure, and flooding. These procedures require the patient to be placed in the phobic situation, such as the setting related to the agoraphobia, and to stay there until he or she is psychologically and emotionally adapted to it. Some patients respond better to flooding whereby they are repeatedly exposed to anxiety-provoking situations, and others to gradual desensitization in which the patient acclimates to one level of a phobic situation before graduating to a more stressful one. Clients can be encouraged to participate in the treatment by choosing their preferred mode. Focusing on small steps in treatment has been found to be rather beneficial to many Caribbean patients. In general, self-exposure is only beneficial to these families after the therapist explains and models the patient's treatment course and teaches/models effective coping strategies (Barlow & Cerny, 1988).

IMPLICATIONS FOR FUTURE RESEARCH

Our review of the current literature on anxiety disorders in Caribbean people has revealed a number of areas in need of further attention. The following is a sample of some of the topics that seem germane to the practicing clinician and would benefit from further clinical research.

1. More qualitative studies of indigenous belief systems.
2. Studies on the efficacy of traditional psychotherapeutic treatments, using Caribbean populations. For example, it should not be assumed that cognitive-behavioral treatment packages developed for panic disorder utilizing white, middle-class Americans will necessarily be effective with clients from different ethnic backgrounds.
3. Studies on attitudes and practices related to the use of antianxiety medications.
4. A close examination of clinical cases in which Caribbean patients presenting with anxiety disorders also continue to seek help from spiritists. How does this affect, help, or hinder the treatment and recovery process?
5. Continued development of acculturation scales and some way of determining patients' satisfaction with their levels of acculturation.
6. More ethnographic studies of culture-bound syndromes.
7. An exploration of the extent to which stereotypes about Caribbean people as "prone to hysteria" and "laid back" may result in either the over- or underdiagnosis of anxiety disorders by clinicians.

REFERENCES

American Psychiatric Association. (1994). *Diagnostic and statistical manual of mental disorders* (4th ed.). Washington, DC: Author.

Aponte, J. F., Young Rivers, R., & Wohl, J. (Eds.). (1995). *Psychological interventions and cultural diversity.* Needham Heights, MA: Allyn & Bacon.

Barlow, D. H., & Cerny, J. A. (1988). *Psychological treatment of panic.* New York: Guilford Press.

Brice, J. (1982). Caribbeans. In M. McGoldrick, J. K. Pearce, & J. Giordano (Eds.), *Ethnicity and family therapy.* New York: Guilford Press.

Brice-Baker, J. (1994). Jamaican women. In L. Comas-Díaz & B. Greene (Eds.), *Women of color: Integrating ethnic and gender indentities in psychotherapy.* New York: Guilford Press.

Boyd-Franklin, N. (1989). *Black families in therapy: A multisystems approach.* New York: Guilford Press.

Burnham, M. A., Hough, R. L., Karno, M., Escobar, J. I., & Telles, C. A. (1987). Acculturation and lifetime prevalence of psychiatric disorders among Mexican Americans in Los Angeles. *Journal of Health and Social Behavior, 28,* 89–102.

Dana, R. H. (1993). *Multicultural assessment perspectives for professional psychology.* Boston: Allyn & Bacon.

Draguns, J. G. (1987). Psychological disorders across cultures. In P. Pedersen (Ed.), *Handbook of cross-cultural counseling and therapy.* New York: Praeger.

Dressler, W. (1985). Stress and sorcery in three social groups. *International Journal of Social Psychiatry, 31*(4), 275–281.

Garcia, M., & Lega, L. I. (1979). Development of a Cuban ethnic identity questionnaire. *Hispanic Journal of the Behavioral Sciences, 1,* 247–261.

Gopaul-McNicol, S. (1993). *Working with West Indian families.* New York: Guilford Press.

Gopaul-McNicol, S. (1995, December). *Treatment of anxiety disorders across cultures: Caribbean families.* Paper presented at the Conference at the Department of Psychiatry St. John's Hospital, Queens, NY.

Griffith, E., Mahy, G., & Young, J. (1986). Psychological benefits of Spiritual Baptist Mourning, II: An empirical assessment. *American Journal of Psychiatry, 143*(2), 404–408.

Kashani, J. H., Beck, N. C., Heoper, E. W., Fallhi, C., Corcoran, C. M., McAllister, J. A., Rosenberg, T. K., & Reid, J. C. (1987). Psychiatric disorders in a community sample of adolescents. *American Journal of Psychiatry, 144,* 584–589.

Kashani, J. H., & Orvaschel, H. (1988). Anxiety disorders in midadolescence: A community sample. *American Journal of Psychiatry, 145,* 960–964.

Kim, S. C. (1985). Family therapy for Asian Americans: A strategic-structural framework. *Psychotherapy, 22,* 342–348.

Marsella, A. J., Kinzie, D., & Gordon, P. (1973). Ethnic variations in the expression of depression. *Journal of Cross-Cultural Psychology, 4,* 435–458.

Mesquite, B., & Frida, N. (1992). Culture variation in emotions: A review. *Psychological Bulletin, 112,* 179–204.

Minuchin, S. (1974). *Families and family therapy.* Cambridge, MA: Harvard University Press.

Murphy, J. (1994). *Working the spirit: Ceremonies of the African diaspora.* Boston: Beacon Press.

New York City Department of Planning, Office of Immigrant Affairs and Population Analysis Division. (1985). *Caribbean immigrants in New York City: A demographic summary.* Unpublished manuscript.

Paniagua, F. A. (1994). *Assessing and treating culturally diverse clients: A practical guide.* Thousand Oaks, CA: Sage.

Ponterotto, J. G., Casas, J. M., Suzuki, L., & Alexander, C. M. (Eds.). (1995). *Handbook of multicultural counseling.* Newbury Park, CA: Sage.

Szapocznik, J., Scopetta, M. A., Arnalde, M., & Kurtines, W. (1978). Cuban value structure: Treatment implications. *Journal of Consulting and Clinical Psychology, 46,* 961–970.

Tseng, W., Xu, D., Ebata, K., Hsu, J., & Cul, Y. (1986). Diagnostic pattern for neuroses among China, Japan and America. *American Journal of Psychiatry, 143,* 1010–1014.

Williams, J. J. (1932). *Voodoos and obeahs: Phases of Caribbean witchcraft.* New York: Dial Press.

6

Asian Americans

GAYLE Y. IWAMASA

Research on the utilization rates of mental health services has shown that Asian Americans underutilize both outpatient and inpatient mental health services, as discussed by Cheung (1991), Zane and Sue (1991), and others. Thus, if experiencing symptoms of an anxiety disorder, an Asian American would be less likely to seek help from a mental health professional, and research has also indicated that Asian Americans who do obtain inpatient mental health services are assigned more severe diagnoses such as psychotic disorders (S. Sue & McKinney, 1975).

Initially, researchers interpreted underutilization of mental health services as an indication that Asian Americans were less likely to experience psychological distress as compared to other ethnic groups. This is an erroneous assumption and, unfortunately, supports the stereotype of Asian Americans as the "model minority." Chan (1991), S. Sue and Morishima (1982), and others have demonstrated that Asian Americans are just as likely as any other ethnic group to experience the stresses of daily living, as well as *added* stress due to discrimination arising from stereotypes and prejudice related to their ethnicity. Several authors have also found that those Asian Americans who do obtain services often suffer from a greater degree of disturbance as compared to European Americans (Brown, Stein, Huang, & Harris, 1973; Durvasula & Sue, 1996; Kinzie & Tseng, 1978). Due to cultural factors, the help of a mental health professional may not be the first choice of Asian Americans when experiencing distress. Thus, it is likely that Asian Americans experience anxiety disorders, and other forms of psychological distress, but either do not seek help or seek help from non-mental health professionals (K. Lin, Inui, Kleinman, & Womack, 1982).

Help seeking among Asian Americans has yet to be examined adequately. However, from whom an Asian American does seek help during times of psychological distress is an important factor for health care professionals and researchers to consider in their work with Asian Americans. Additionally, as will be discussed in more detail later in this chapter, there is evidence that some Asian Americans may manifest symptoms of anxiety differently than conventional symptoms of anxiety as defined by Western mental health professionals.

Before we discuss the expression of anxiety symptoms and treatment issues for Asian Americans, we must first address the question "Who are Asian Americans?" Unfortunately, this question does not have a simple answer. Although many believe it is easy to identify an Asian American individual by his or her appearance, and thus make certain assumptions about that individual, the heterogeneity among the various Asian ethnic groups in the United States is staggering.

WHO ARE ASIAN AMERICANS?

The 1990 U.S. Census indicated that approximately 3% of the population was Asian American/Pacific Islander (U.S. Bureau of the Census, 1992). The Census Bureau also reported that, as a collective group, Asian Americans are one of the fastest growing ethnic and cultural groups in the United States.

When we discuss Asian Americans, one of the biggest problems, in general and in the published mental health literature, is the assumption of homogeneity—the idea that all Asian Americans are alike; that each Asian American will experience and report distress in the same way. When we use the term "Asian Americans," we are classifying over 25 ethnic groups into one category based on their common heritage in Asia and the Pacific Islands, on their similar appearance, and on their cultural values. In the next sections, the similarities and differences in cultural characteristics among the various Asian American ethnic groups will be discussed.

Whereas many clinicians may feel knowledgeable about the Asian ethnic groups who have had a long history in the United States, such as Japanese Americans and Chinese Americans, many clinicians are probably not as familiar with the history of other, smaller Asian ethnic groups who have immigrated more recently to the United States such as Filipinos, Vietnamese Americans, Hmong, Cambodians, Thais, Laotians, and so forth. Each ethnic group has a distinct history, both in their original country and also in terms of their reasons for immigrating to the United States, their familiarity with American values and customs, the immigration process, and their adaptation experiences once arriving in the United States. In addition, the huge number of bi-ethnic individuals who have one Asian parent and a parent of another ethnicity also must be considered. Clinicians may be familiar with the term "Amerasian," which was first popularized at the end of the Vietnam war, when many children of U.S. servicemen and Vietnamese women were born. Individuals from each of these groups share characteristics that are similar, but also possess characteristics that make them different from one another. Just as those having Irish, German, English, or Polish ancestry may be similar in some ways, yet clearly different in other ways, individuals from diverse Asian ethnic and cultural backgrounds should also be appreciated as possessing unique cultural characteristics, values, and traditions.

Between- and Within-Group Similarities

Clearly, many Asian ethnic groups share common physical characteristics and cultural values, which sometimes erroneously leads others to assume that Asian Americans are a homogeneous group of people. In the worst cases, stereotypes of Asian Americans are developed and reinforced when individuals *only* attend to those characteristics that group people together, rather than focusing on those characteristics that distinguish one individual from another. Although this section focuses on similarities among the various Asian ethnic groups, clinicians must be cognizant of the fact that the clients they are working with in treatment must be viewed as individuals, and as with all group characteristics, may vary in the degree to which they adhere to the following characteristics.

Focus on Family

In many Asian ethnic groups, the needs of the family take precedence over the individual's needs (Ayelsworth, Ossorio, & Osaki, 1980; Kim, 1980; Kitano & Kikumura, 1976; Lyman, 1974; Morales, 1974; Petersen, 1978; Shu & Satele, 1977). F. L. K. Hsu (1971) described how Chinese culture stresses that bonds between family members be continuous, resulting in the individual being "rooted" in his or her immediate family, even if the person moves a long distance from the family. This is in contrast to Western culture, which emphasizes individuality and encourages the individual to branch out from the family and plant his or her own roots. Hsu argued that, in Chinese families, affective and emotional needs are to be met within the family. Thus, conformity to the wishes of the family is seen as crucial. As a result, guilt and shame are often used as powerful means of control, as compared to the external measures of control often used in Western families (Chew & Ogi, 1987; Payton, 1985).

In many Asian American families, one's behavior is not only a reflection of the self, but of the entire family. Thus, the consequences for experiencing distress are not only personal, but encompass all family members. Interdependence among family members is valued, thus clinicians should not necessarily pathologize such an attachment to, and dependence on, family members among Asian Americans. As a result of this interdependence, divorce and separation rates among Asian Americans are very low, as is the number of elderly Asian Americans who live alone or in nursing facilities. In many Asian American families, each member has a specific position in the family hierarchy based on age and sex (Ho, 1990; Strom, Park, & Daniels, 1987). Those who are older and who are male assume a higher status level. It is often expected that as family members become elderly, they will most likely remain in the home of the eldest son's immediate family.

Focus on Community

The focus on the "group" as opposed to the individual often extends to the community as a whole. While Asian American families are very cohesive, the role of the extended family and community is also important. The reputation one's family has within the community and the contributions the family makes to the community are often the focus of many Asian American families' activities. Such activities are integral to the well-being of the community and ensure its survival. One can get a feel for the strong sense of community among these ethnic enclaves by visiting the various "Chinatowns" or "Little Tokyos" around the United States. Newer Asian immigrants, such as those from Korea and Vietnam, have also tended to settle in areas where they are near others of their own ethnic heritage, such as the Hmong in Minneapolis and Vietnamese in Oklahoma City. These communities tend to be close-knit, and members are expected to rely on and support each other.

Emphasis on Religion/Spirituality

Individuals within the various Asian ethnic groups ascribe to many different religions, and religion and spirituality are often deeply embedded in everyday family life. Attendance at religious services and participation in activities sponsored by the church are often important community events, promoting cohesiveness and instilling pride in traditional cultural practices. Additionally, church elders often serve as unofficial community leaders, as well as mediators in conflicts that cannot be solved from within or between families. As such, church elders often serve as mental health paraprofessionals in Asian American communities (Choy, 1979; Hurh & Kim, 1984; Kim, 1980; Kim-Goh, 1993).

Respect for Elders

Elderly individuals are considered experienced and wise, and are often viewed with reverence (Anderson, 1983). This is quite different than the Western "fear" of getting old. As indicated earlier, elderly Asian Americans often remain in the homes of their children to form multigenerational families, rather than being placed alone in convalescent homes. When decisions must be made, the grandparents' opinions often carry more weight than those of other family members. Among children, respect for parents and other authority figures is emphasized (Uba, 1994).

Emphasis on Hard Work and Education

Academic and occupational success are often very important to many Asian Americans. Such success is believed to be an indication of the family's and community's support of the person (Kalish & Moriwaki, 1973; Payton, 1985; S. Sue & Sue, 1973). Thus, the status not only of the person, but also of the family and larger community, is elevated. In selecting a career, the family's wishes, particularly those of the adults' and grandparents', may supersede those of the individual. Parents often not only expect their children to obtain high grades, but also to receive higher education (Chia, 1989; C. Lin & Fu, 1990; Sollenberger, 1968; Yao, 1985). Acceptance of delayed gratification while attending school or in training is also common (Young, 1972). Even though parental high expectations place great pressures on Asian American children to succeed, they often do not receive much overt praise when they do well (Nagata, 1989), nor do they get as much pedagogical assistance from their parents (Hess, Chang, & McDevitt, 1987). Thus, Asian American children are expected to do well, yet may not get much assistance, praise, or credit for their accomplishments.

Communication Style

Research has indicated that communication patterns of many Asian Americans differ from those of European Americans. Several studies have found lower frequency of verbalization among Asian Americans, both in the home and in social situations (Uba, 1994). Uba postulated several explanations for this: (1) Asian Americans might have higher levels of inhibition; (2) Asian Americans may rely more on nonverbal rather than verbal communication (Johnson, Marsella, & Johnson, 1974; Yu & Kim, 1983); (3) emphasis on being deferential to authority may limit verbal communication (Tsui & Schultz, 1988); (4) well-defined roles may result in less need for direct verbal communication (Tsui & Schultz, 1988); (5) due to the "model minority" stereotype, some Asian Americans may inadvertently be rewarded for less verbal behaviors and punished for being verbal (D. W. Sue, 1989; Fort, Watts, & Lesser, 1969); and (6) children of immigrants and of later generations are less likely to speak in Asian languages in the home, thus reducing the amount of conversation.

Another aspect of communication among many Asian Americans is restraint in emotional expressiveness (McDermott et al., 1984). Asian cultural values emphasize self-control and interpersonal harmony on a continual basis, rather than demonstrating affection openly and for specific reasons. Asian American parents are more likely to express their affection and love for their children in indirect ways (e.g., sacrificing for their children) rather than through words, hugs, or kisses (Shon & Ja, 1982).

Interpersonal Harmony and Cooperation

Traditional Asian values of cooperation and avoidance of conflict are sometimes interpreted as conformity and lack of assertiveness. Indeed, research has indicated that some Asian Americans score higher on conformity (Hsu, Tseng, Ashton, McDermott, & Char, 1985; Sollenberger, 1968; S. Sue & Morishima, 1982) and lower on assertiveness (Fukuyama & Greenfield, 1983) as compared to European Americans. These results must be interpreted with caution, however, as several Asian American researchers have obtained results showing that responses to self-report measures and behavioral observations are not highly correlated (D. Sue, Ino, & Sue, 1983; D. Sue, Sue, & Ino, 1990; Zane, Sue, Hu, & Kwon, 1991). Asian Americans will often report low assertiveness on self-report measures, but behavioral observation measures have indicated that Asian Americans can *behave* assertively in certain situations (Yi, Zane, & Sue, 1986).

Sex Roles

Stereotypes often reflect the notion that Asian American men and women ascribe to traditional sex roles. Traditional Asian cultures are patriarchal and sex roles tend to be clearly differentiated (Lee & Cynn, 1991; Miller, Reynolds, & Cambra, 1987; D. W. Sue, 1989). As indicated earlier, in many Asian American families, elders and males have more prestige within the family. These roles are believed to provide the balance necessary to achieve equilibrium (Yang, 1991). As can be expected, adherence to traditional Asian sex roles varies greatly among Asian Americans, particularly among those individuals who are more acculturated. Such shifts in adherence to traditional sex roles are likely to be more pronounced among women. Women with higher levels of acculturation may be less likely to ascribe to traditional Asian sex roles and behaviors.

Between- and Within-Group Differences

Although there exist numerous similarities across and between the various Asian ethnic groups, between- and within-group differences are frequently ignored. Some may acknowledge the existence of between-group differences, but within-group differences are also important and highlight the need to view clients as individuals. For example, a first generation Japanese American is quite different in a number of ways from a fourth generation Japanese American. The following list of characteristics is by no means comprehensive. Rather, it merely serves to highlight some of the individual differences that clinicians should consider in their work with, and conceptualization of, Asian American clients.

Ethnic Identity

Ethnic identity is often defined as a person's sense of belonging to an ethnic group based on shared ethnic characteristics (Phinney, 1990; Shibutani & Kwan, 1965). It can be a part of a person's self-concept, or it can be how others categorize a person. Although, it is beyond the scope of this chapter to summarize all of the literature on ethnic identity in general, and Asian American identity in particular, Uba's (1994) conceptualization of Asian American ethnic identity will be summarized. She distinguishes between three aspects of Asian American ethnic identity: (1) consciousness of ethnicity, (2) adoption of an ethnic identity, and (3) application of that ethnic identity. Ethnic consciousness is thought to include both "ideological ethnicity" (knowledge of the group's customs and beliefs) and "behavioral ethnicity" (knowledge of behavioral norms in interpersonal interactions). Adoption of an ethnic identity involves incorporation of ethnically based behavior patterns, values, and beliefs into one's sense of self, and feeling in some way connected to other members of the ethnic group. Uba argues that this is not an all-or-nothing phenomenon; some individuals may strongly identify with many aspects of their ethnic group, while others may only mildly do so. Application of one's ethnic identity entails having a schema for an Asian American ethnic identity, which is activated at various times depending on the situation the individual is in. In this sense, it is dynamic rather than static. Thus, at times ethnic identity might be invoked along with other types of identities, while at other times, only non-ethnically based identities will be activated.

Uba (1994) emphasizes that the diversity in ethnic identity among Asian Americans may be due to a number of factors such as racism, immigrant/refugee experiences, difficulty with integrating several ethnicities, misidentification by others (e.g., being viewed as Japanese rather than as Japanese American), and the desire for individuality. Asian Americans will vary in their experiences with racist comments and behaviors, in how they can balance several different cultural values, and in their desire to be seen as individuals. Thus, assuming that all Asian Americans have the same level of ethnic identity would be erroneous.

Language

Just as there are numerous different Asian ethnic groups, there are even more Asian languages. Even what we often refer to as "Chinese" is actually comprised of numerous different dialects, for example, Cantonese and Mandarin, each with their own terminology and grammatical rules. Thus, one should not assume that an individual who speaks one Chinese dialect will automatically understand another dialect. In addition, there are many within-group and between-group differences in facility with the English language. Obviously, an Asian American immigrant may not have the same English-speaking capability as a third-generation Asian American. One should also not assume that a later-generation Asian American individual speaks, reads, or understands the language of his or her ancestry.

Acculturation/Generational Status/Immigration Status

Acculturation may be defined as the process of adopting the values and customs of the dominant society. It has been examined as one of the major within-group difference variables among Asian Americans. The Suinn-Lew Asian Self-Identity Acculturation Scale (SL-ASIA; Suinn, Rickland-Figueroa, Lew, & Vigil, 1987) is currently the only scale available to assess level of acculturation among Asian Americans, and thus has been used in much of the empirical literature on Asian Americans. It is a 21-item self-report questionnaire that yields a total acculturation score. Some argue that the unidimensional aspect of the SL-ASIA does not fully express the complexity of a multidimensional construct of acculturation (Iwamasa, 1996) and that clinicians should not make assumptions about one's ethnic identity or adherence to cultural values and traditions based on one score. However, the SL-ASIA is useful as an initial screening of acculturation level and can assist the clinician in developing additional questions about the client's personal history.

A major way in which Asian Americans differ both within and between the various ethnic groups is in generational status. Those who are born in the United States (second generation or later) are American citizens and may have a different perspective on their ethnic heritage as compared to immigrants, refugees, or first-generation Asian Americans. Generational status also may influence the acculturation process. Iwamasa (1996) found that foreign-born Asian Americans had lower levels of acculturation as compared to U.S.-born Asian Americans.

Immigration status is also an important variable to consider. The various Asian immigrant groups have had very diverse immigration experiences. Some individuals left their countries willingly, while others felt forced to leave. Some individuals have a better standard of living in the United States, while others have a lower standard of living than what they were used to in their home countries. Some individuals came to the United States as refugees, with few or no financial resources, whereas other immigrants were prominent members of their community in their home country before coming to the United States and were able to bring financial resources with them. Some individuals, such as Filipinos, have had extensive experience and familiarity with traditional American culture, as compared to others with little familiarity of the United States before immigrating. All of these issues will greatly impact how the individual adjusts to his or her new environment. Sensitivity to these experiences are important in terms of interpreting an individual's distress.

Religion

It is believed that Confucianism, Taoism, and Buddhism underlie many traditional Asian values. Many of the traditional Asian cultural values discussed earlier, such as interpersonal harmony; the quest for knowledge; the importance of fulfilling obligations, particularly to one's family; the precedence of the group over the individual; and so forth, are believed to have been founded in such religions. As indicated earlier, various Asian ethnic groups adhere to various religions. For example, although one might assume that a Japanese American individual is Buddhist, he or she is equally likely to adhere to some form of Christianity.

Cultural Traditions

Each ethnic group has its own cultural traditions and practices. As mentioned previously, many of these cultural traditions and celebrations are based in religious beliefs. Some Asian Americans may celebrate the same holidays as European Americans, but with different traditions. New Year's Eve, for instance, often celebrated among European Americans by toasting champagne, is celebrated by many Japanese Americans by drinking *ozoni* soup. The soup is made with soft rice cakes and seaweed and is thought to bring good luck. For many Chinese Americans, the new year is also a major event to be celebrated; however, their new year does not fall on January 1.

It is also important to recognize that traditions specific to some Asian American groups might have originated from the United States and not from the country of ethnic heritage. For example, Japanese Americans developed *Nisei Week*, which is held yearly to celebrate the accomplishments of *niseis*, or second-generation Japanese Americans, as well as to remember traditional Japanese customs and events.

Sex Roles

There has not been much research on sex roles among Asian Americans, and what research has been conducted has yielded equivocal results. As indicated earlier, sex roles in many Asian cultures are more clearly differentiated than in Western cultures. This needs to be tempered by knowledge about adherence to traditional family roles, as well as by the individual's generational, educational, and occupational status. For example, an immigrant Chinese woman who was raised in a family that subscribed more strictly to traditional family values will be more likely to adhere to traditional sex roles than would a fourth-generation Chinese American woman who was raised in a family without such an emphasis on traditional sex roles. For further elaboration on the historical experiences of Asian American women, the reader is encouraged to consult Bradshaw (1994) and Tien (1994).

Education Level/Occupational Status/ Socioeconomic Status

Although many people believe in the "model minority" stereotype and assume that all Asian Americans are highly educated, have high-paying jobs, and a high level of income, the fact is that there is a great deal of diversity in educational, occupational, and socioeconomic levels among Asian Americans (Almirol, 1990; Cabezas, Shinagawa, & Kawaguchi, 1990). In summarizing the changes in trends of the educational and income status of Asian Americans in recent years, Chan (1991) also emphasizes that statistics used to support the "model minority" stereotype have often been interpreted erroneously. For example, although it was argued in the past that many Asian American groups had higher income per family as compared to other ethnic groups, reports frequently would neglect to mention that Asian American families also typically had more individuals employed and contributing to family income as compared to European American families, and that Asian Americans with advanced degrees earned far less than their European American counterparts. Additionally, many Asian Americans tend to live in urban areas where the cost of living is high. Chan also underscores that one of the problems with making sweeping statements about the current socioeconomic status of Asian Americans is that scholars have used different models in developing their studies and in interpreting their data.

Some Asian ethnic groups have managed to do well in the United States in spite of historical institutional racism. The level of education among those groups who have a long history in the United States, such as Chinese Americans and Japanese Americans, is fairly high. However, the educational level among some of the newer immigrant groups is not as high. This is likely due to economic and language problems often facing immigrants, as well as the current trend of decreased tolerance in providing quality education to immigrant children.

Age

While examination of the distribution of Asian Americans across various age ranges indicates a bimodal distribution, in general the Asian American population is a relatively young one (U.S. Bureau of the Census, 1992). Most Asian Americans are of school age or between the ages of 22 and 59. Adolescents and older adults are less frequent among Asian Americans. The 1990 regional breakdown by age is as follows: In the Northeast region, Asian Americans comprised 2.6% of the population, with the majority of Asian Americans being adults; in the Midwest and Southern regions, Asian Americans comprised 1.3% of the population, with bimodal distributions similar to the overall U.S. age distribution; in the Western region, Asian Americans comprised 7.7% of the population, the majority of Asian Americans being adults. In addition, the age distribution of Asian Americans with longer histories of being in the United States (such as Japanese Americans and

Chinese Americans) tends to be more varied as compared to the age range among more recent Asian immigrant groups, such as Vietnamese, Hmong, and Laotians, who tend to be much younger.

In summary, when conducting clinical work with Asian Americans, it is important to understand general group characteristics, as well as the unique characteristics and qualities that one's client may bring to the therapy setting. The therapist's level of competence (or incompetence) may significantly impact the well-being of the client. Problems of misdiagnosis due to ignorance, as well as mistreatment of clients, is not only possible but has occurred, with very dire consequences. In S. Sue and Morishima's (1982) book, they present a 1979 newspaper article that described a Chinese-speaking man who was incarcerated in an Illinois state mental hospital for 25 years. The article indicated that physicians described the man as incoherent and unintelligible, and thus gave him a diagnosis of psychosis. The article also stated that he was placed in restraints at times, because he would attempt to visit the only other Chinese-speaking patient in the hospital. We all assume that progress in cultural sensitivity in mental health services has been made over the past 16 years. The next section reviews the recent research on anxiety disorders among Asian Americans.

SUMMARY OF RESEARCH

There are many gaps in the research on anxiety disorders and Asian Americans. The research does not fully cover the various ethnic groups, nor does it cover the entire spectrum of anxiety disorders. Few researchers have examined the epidemiology of anxiety disorders in Asian Americans, let alone other psychiatric disorders. Additionally, one of the problems with the literature is that it is difficult to know at times whether or not anxiety, depression, or general psychological distress is being measured. The following areas will be reviewed in this section: assessment issues, anxiety disorders among Asian American immigrants, factors affecting the development of anxiety symptoms, and culture-specific anxiety disorders.

Assessment Issues

Before epidemiology issues are explored, assessment issues must first be examined. The reader is encouraged to review Guarnaccia's discussion of overall concerns regarding assessment issues across cultures (see Chapter 1). The following section focuses specifically on Asian American populations.

One cannot assume that the definition of anxiety as indicated in the fourth edition of the *Diagnostic and Statistical Manual of Mental Disorders* (DSM-IV; American Psychiatric Association, 1994) or *International Classification of Diseases—Ninth Revision* (U.S. Department of Health and Human Services, 1991) is how Asian Americans define anxiety. In Hawaii, Takeuchi, Kuo, Kim, and Leaf (1989) factor analyzed the Symptom Checklist 90 (SCL-90) with a sample of three Asian ethnic groups, Filipinos, Japanese Americans, and Native Hawaiians, and European Americans. The SCL-90, one of the most frequently used scales to assess various dimensions of psychological distress, contains five factors, one of which is purported to assess anxiety, and was developed on a predominantly European American sample. Takeuchi and his colleagues found that the original factor structure of the scale did not work with the Filipinos, Japanese Americans, and Native Hawaiians. The researchers reported that interpreting the SCL-90 as suggested by the scale developers did not differentiate between somatization and general distress for these groups. Their study indicated that the Asian ethnic groups tended to include other psychological items in the factor that purportedly assessed somatic complaints.

This research points to some important issues to keep in mind when treating Asian Americans clients; somatic complaints may possibly be higher or more pronounced in anxiety disorders and other psychological distress. These results point to the importance of health care workers understanding how culture might influence the reporting of symptoms. Takeuchi et al. (1989) recommended that, in their initial and ongoing assessment of Asian American clients, clinicians should attempt to differentiate between general psychological distress and somatization. Thus, clinicians should not only assess typical anxiety symptoms, but also assess somatic symptoms as well.

Imada (1989) investigated the connotative meanings of anxiety, fear, and depression in a Japanese sample. He found that experiences of *fu-an* (anxiety) were found to be more similar to those of *yu-utsu* (depression) than to those of *kyo-fu* (fear). This is in contrast to previous research with American participants who equate anxiety symptoms with fear rather than depression. In fact, with his Japanese participants, Imada found that experiences of *fu-an* overlapped little with Western definitions of anxiety and emphasized physical symptoms more. Furthermore, he found that his participants rated experiences of *fu-an* as more distressing and more ambiguous than experiences of anxiety. This research highlights how generational status and acculturation of Asian Americans might influence one's conceptualization symptoms, that is, there may be some major differences in the interpretation of symptoms between first generation and later-generation Japanese Americans.

Finally, Tseng, Asai, Kitanishi, McLaughlin, and Kyomen (1992) found cultural differences in how Japanese and American psychiatrists diagnose social phobia. They showed both groups of psychiatrists videotapes and written case histories of four Japanese clients and two Japanese American clients who were clinically diagnosed with social phobia in their respective countries. The Japanese psychiatrists were highly consistent in their diagnoses of social phobia of the Japanese clients, but not of the Japanese American clients. The American psychiatrists were not consistent in their application of diagnoses for either the Japanese or Japanese American clients. The authors suggested that social phobia may be a more common occurrence in Japan as compared to the United States and cited that social phobia was not included in the DSM classification system until 1980. Thus, they suggested that Japanese psychiatrists are likely to have more familiarity with the disorder than American psychiatrists. As will be reviewed in more detail later in this chapter, the Japanese classification system for social phobia, known as *taijin kyofusho*, is much more elaborate, with four different subtypes. This research highlights the importance of cultural differences in the interpretation and meaning of symptoms during assessment. Even though in the United States, clinicians might interpret symptoms to be indicative of a certain disorder, the client, particularly if an immigrant, might have a different conceptualization of the symptoms.

The results of the above study support the contention of numerous authors who emphasize that cultural considerations must be included when assessing and treating Asian American clients (Chin, 1983; Flaskerud & Akutsu, 1993; Flaskerud & Hu, 1992). From a behavioral perspective, Tanaka-Matsumi, Seiden, and Lam (1996) suggest a "culturally informed functional analysis," or CIFA, that incorporates the clients' interpretation and meaning of his or her symptoms into the assessment process. The argument is that such an analysis will lead to treatment interventions that more closely match the client's interpretation of symptoms; thus, treatment compliance will be improved and treatment will be more efficacious.

Anxiety Disorders among Asian Immigrants

One aspect of anxiety disorders among Asian Americans that has received perhaps the most attention from mental health researchers is the incidence of anxiety disorders (particularly posttraumatic stress disorder) among recent Asian immigrants. It is beyond the scope of this chapter to summarize all of the research on anxiety disorders among Asian immigrants. Readers interested in obtaining a more thorough review of the literature on psychological trauma among Asian immigrants are encouraged to consult Abueg and Chun (1996), Chan (1991), Hinton et al. (1993), Tran (1993), and Uba (1994). However, a few aspects of the literature will be highlighted here for clinicians to consider in their work with Asian immigrant clients.

Most clinicians are aware that the most recent Asian immigrants to the United States are primary candidates for developing anxiety symptoms. The stress of leaving one's country, although often war torn and filled with economic strife, the stress of leaving family members behind, and the stress of miserable traveling conditions (think of the "boat people" and what it was like for them, as well as the recent Chinese immigrants who lived like sardines while traveling here in ships and boats) all occur before the individuals even arrive in the United States. Once Asian immigrants arrive here, they are often confronted with poor living conditions, poor access to medical attention, poor access to employment opportunities, and insensitive and possibly racist people who are not willing to be patient or helpful to those who look different, speak a different language, or speak English with an accent. One can easily see how the development of anxiety and depressive symptoms is possible. Typical symptoms include nightmares and decreased sense of personal efficacy (Tran, 1993), increased sense of marginality (Smither & Rodriguez-Giegling, 1979), pain, demoralization, anger, and worry (Kroll et al., 1989).

Several researchers have recognized the need for more culturally appropriate assessment tools. Mollica, Wyshak, de Marneffe, Khuon, and Lavelle (1987) developed and validated Cambodian, Laotian, and Vietnamese language versions of the Hopkins Symptom Checklist 25. Beiser and Fleming (1986) also developed assessment measures for Southeast Asian refugees who relocated to British Columbia. They reported that the scales, which measure panic, depression, somatization, and well-being, demonstrated good reliability, concurrent validity, and stability across several samples.

With the Vietnamese language version of the Hopkins Symptom Checklist 25, Felsman, Leong, Johnson, and Felsman (1990) examined three subgroups of Vietnamese refugees: unaccompanied minors, adolescents, and young adults. They found high levels of anxiety among all three groups and self-report of poor health status. They also found high levels of depression among the young adult group. Some of the stressors specific to these groups that were believed to influence these results include living apart from their families, lack of adult guidance, and an uncontrollable and unpredictable environment.

There is evidence that some of the anxiety symptoms experienced by Asian immigrants and refugees abate over time, as the immigrant begins to adapt to his or her new environment. Westermeyer, Neider, and Vang (1984) examined Hmong refugees at 1.5 years and 3.5 years postmigration. Using a translated version of the SCL-90, they found that their sample of 89 nonclinical participants improved their scores on the following subscales from the first assessment to the second: somatization, obsessive–compulsiveness, interpersonal sensitivity, and phobic anxiety. They did not compare their sample's scores with those of the SCL-90 standardization group, so it is not clear whether or not initial scores were different from those of the standardization sample. However, Westermeyer and his colleagues suggested that the psychological state of the immigrants may have improved as they learned to adapt to their new environment. Although their study was correlational, thus causality cannot be determined, it was found that ability to obtain employment, proficiency with the English language, and integration into the new community were related to lower scores at the second assessment. This research highlights the hope that anxiety symptoms may decrease over time, but should sensitize clinicians working with recent immigrants to assess the severity of anxiety symptoms carefully and to implement practical treatment interventions that will directly address the needs of the client. The client may benefit from information about English language classes, job skills training, and encouragement to develop relationships with other immigrants (both new and old), as well as making connections with nonimmigrants in the community.

Again, this brief section should not substitute for a more thorough review of the literature on anxiety symptoms and disorders among Asian immigrants. However, it serves to highlight some of the stressors likely to be experienced by these individuals. Clinicians must be aware of such factors when assessing and working with immigrants, in order to implement interventions that will specifically address the experiences that lead to the development of anxiety symptoms.

Factors Affecting the Development of Anxiety Symptoms

The emphasis on community and family in Asian culture may actually serve as a protective factor against the development of some anxiety symptoms. N. Lin, Ensel, Simeone, and Kuo (1979) found that social support was significantly and negatively related to illness symptoms in a Chinese American sample in Washington, DC. Given that family and community are important Asian cultural values, this may actually work to decrease the development of anxiety and other distress symptoms in Asian Americans. This highlights one of the resources available to health care providers—using family and community to support treatment.

However, as indicated earlier, some aspects about traditional Asian values might also increase the likelihood of the development of an anxiety disorder. As discussed earlier, Tseng et al. (1992) reported that the incidence of social phobia was higher in Japan as compared to the United States and, further, that four subtypes of social phobia were included in the Japanese mental disorder classification system. These authors also noted the emphasis on sensitivity and concern about social interactions and relationships: "Because Japanese behavior is sensitive to situational variation, especially the boundary between, within, and without the intimate situation, a person is naturally cautious about his exposure to the outside world. The Japanese must control their behavior to conform to situationally prescribed codes of conduct" (p. 381). Such values may increase the likelihood of developing and exacerbating social-phobic symptoms in an individual who lacks adequate coping skills. Originally thought to be a Japanese-specific set of symptoms, *taijin kyofusho* is now believed to occur in Korea and China as well.

Finally, as indicated in the previous section on anxiety symptoms and Asian immigrants, one can see how the immigration experience, as well as the immigrant's resources to adapt to his or her new environment, might affect the development of anxiety symptoms.

Specific Cultural Interpretations of Anxiety

Hwa-Byung

K. Lin (1983) described three cases of *hwa-byung*, a Korean folk illness experienced by patients and their families to be a physical affliction, despite the fact that its manifestations include both physiological and psychological symptoms. From a Western perspective, *hwa-byung* appears to be a mixture of depression and anxiety. In addition, the patient often recognizes interpersonal conflicts and anger as precipitating factors to the somatic complaints. Each patient described by K. Lin also identified an epigastric mass that was not identified on physical examination. Symptoms of the disorder included: (1) repressed or suppressed anger of long duration; (2) various somatic complaints (e.g., panic attacks, psychomotor retardation, tiredness, loss of appetite, weight loss, indigestion, dizziness, insomnia); (3) feelings of helplessness, resentfulness, and guilt; (4) tension; (5) pressure or compression in the epigastrium; and (6) fear of impending death despite medical reassurance. With these patients, antidepressants were prescribed, and with two of the patients, supportive psychotherapy also was utilized. Lin reported these treatments as being effective in treating the symptoms.

K. Lin followed up his initial report with several colleagues in 1992. They interviewed 109 Korean Americans, ages 18 years and older, living in the metropolitan Los Angeles area. Out of the 109 subjects, 13 (11.9%) reported having suffered from *hwa-byung*. In this study, Lin and colleagues conceptualized the disorder to be more closely related to major depression. However, this apparently culture-specific disorder is presented here so that clinicians are aware of how both the physiological and psychological symptoms of *hwa-byung* may be interpreted by Korean American clients. It also emphasizes how culture plays an important role in the experience of symptoms, and how Western classification systems may not be appropriate in terms of understanding the experience and expression of distress. Understanding of the presentation of such symptoms is also important for the clinician, particularly due to the general difficulty clinicians often have in differentiating between depressive and anxiety symptoms.

Taijin Kyofusho

As summarized earlier, Tseng et al. (1992) found differences in how Japanese and American psychiatrists conceptualized phobic symptoms. The following is a more detailed discussion of *taijin kyofusho,* which has been described by Kirmayer (1991) as the Japanese equivalent of what U.S. mental health professionals refer to as social phobia. DSM-IV (American Psychiatric Association, 1994) describes social phobia as marked and persistent fear of one or more social or performance situations in which the person is exposed to unfamiliar people or scrutiny by others. The individual fears he or she will act in a humiliating or embarrassing way. Exposure to the feared social situation provokes anxiety; thus the situation is avoided.

Taijin kyofusho is described in Japan as a "neurotic disorder characterized by 'the presence of extraordinary intense anxiety and tension in social settings with others, a fear of being looked down upon by others, making others feel unpleasant, and being disliked by others, so that it leads to withdrawal from or avoidance of social relations' " (Kasahara, 1975, cited in Tseng et al., 1992, p. 380). Some of the factors that might lead to the intense anxiety are concerns about blushing, emitting offensive odors, staring inappropriately, and improper facial expressions. An individual might not actually be doing these behaviors, but instead, the anxiety is a result of the fear that others perceive that he or she is engaging in the behaviors. In most incidences, individuals describe a single circumscribed fear.

Kleinknecht, Dinnel, Tanouye-Wilson, and Lonner (1994) summarized the differences between *taijin kyofusho* and social phobia. Although there are many similarities, some forms of *taijin kyofusho* appear to correspond more closely with DSM-IV categories of body dysmorphic disorder, personality disorders, and even delusional disorders. Whereas Western conceptualizations differentiate these groups of symptoms, the Japanese conceptualization includes the various types of *taijin kyofusho* as being a single disorder with a continuum of severity. The four subtypes of *taijin kyofusho* are (1) transient type (temporary, usually occurs in adolescents); (2) neurotic type; (3) severe type, which often includes delusions or ideas of reference; and (4) secondary type, which is a phobia that occurs concomitantly with schizophrenia. Mori and Kitanishi (1984, cited in Tseng et al., 1992) found that Japanese psychiatrists were most likely to equate the DSM diagnosis of social phobia with the neurotic type of *taijin kyofusho*.

Kleinknecht et al. described the major difference between social phobia and *taijin kyofusho* as being the focus of the social anxiety. With social phobia, anxiety is due to concern that the person will embarrass *him- or herself*. With *taijin kyofusho*, the concern is that the person will do something that will offend or embarrass *others*. As discussed earlier, traditional Asian cultural values emphasize the importance of the group over the individual. One can see how this emphasis on interpersonal relations among the Japanese could result in intense anxiety in those who might lack adequate coping skills or who have low levels of self-confidence. Thus, one might experience anxiety symptoms as a result of the cultural emphasis on interpersonal harmony.

In summary, more research on anxiety disorders and Asian Americans is needed. Although the studies described above highlight the importance of cultural considerations in the assessment and treatment of Asian Americans, we need more empirical data on the conceptualization, experiences, and expression of anxiety symptoms among Asian Americans. When we have a better understanding of such issues, we can then begin to address the development of culturally appropriate interventions for Asian Americans and training programs for health care professionals who work with Asian American clients. Until then, how can mental health professional provide appropriate services to Asian Americans with anxiety problems? The following section provides some suggestions.

WORKING WITH ASIAN AMERICANS

From Whom Do Asian Americans with Anxiety Symptoms Seek Help?

Given the research that indicates that most Asian Americans do not seek mental health services when experiencing distress, from whom are Asian Americans most likely to seek assistance? Although there are no hard data, primary care and general practitioner physicians are most likely to be seen when physical and somatic symptoms are predominant. Some Asian Americans might also seek the assistance of clergy, or spiritual leaders, if they perceive that their symptoms are spiritual in origin. Due to the strong ties to family and community, it is also logical to assume that many Asian Americans in distress would turn to their immediate family, or to another respected family member or community leader for assistance. As discussed earlier, level of acculturation also likely influences help-seeking behaviors among Asian Americans.

The fact that many Asian Americans are reluctant to seek assistance from a mental health professional when experiencing distress makes the task of providing culturally appropriate mental health services challenging. One of the aspects that the field of mental health needs to examine then, is how well we are doing in addressing the mental health needs of Asian Americans? This question can be examined in two ways. One is to view it from a structural or institutional level. The other is to view it from the perspective of an individual mental health professional working either in the context of a large institution or in a private or group practice. In either case, mental health professionals must address the types of services they are providing and conduct periodic assessments to ensure an appropriate standard of care for their Asian American clients.

Addressing Barriers to Culturally Appropriate Treatment at the Institutional Level

In order to address the question of how well the mental health profession is doing in terms of providing culturally appropriate mental health services for Asian Americans, hospitals, clinics, and directors or administrators of such facilities can ask and answer the following questions. Although not a complete list of questions, it will at least provide facilities with guidelines for evaluating whether or not the facility is doing what it could to promote the mental health of Asian Americans.

1. *Are services accessible to the Asian American community?* Hospital and clinic administrators should assess whether or not the Asian American community is aware of the services provided by the facility. Do people in the community know about various screenings and evaluations that the clinic or hospital offers? What is attendance like at these types of community service events? How does the facility advertise such services to the community? Does the facility offer hours that are convenient to those in the community, such as evening hours? Many individuals work during the day (often longer than a typical 8-hour workday), and are not able to make appointments during the

day. How good a job does the facility do in making its services accessible to the community? For example, is the fee structure afford-able to most members of the community, particularly those who might not have health insurance? Does the facility offer outreach services to the community? In other words, does the facility bring services to the community as opposed to expecting the community to come to them?

2. *Does the facility make an effort to recruit ethnically diverse staff?* One obvious sign of commitment to providing culturally appropriate ser-vices is to have a staff that reflects diversity. Asian Americans who are aware that there are Asian American staff members at the facility might be more likely to obtain services at that facility.

3. *Are there staff members who speak a variety of languages?* As with an ethnically diverse staff, having staff members who speak the lan-guage of the client is an obvious sign of commitment to culturally appropriate treatment. This is particularly important in areas where there are large numbers of recent Asian immigrants and refugees. If a client does not feel understood, or is actually not understood, by the clinician, he or she is less likely to return for follow-up appointments or be compliant with treatment recommendations.

4. *Does the facility support and emphasize the importance of cultural sensitivity?* This may be reflected in staff development activities such as bringing in guest speakers with expertise in working with Asian American clients; paying for staff to attend workshops focusing on issues of diversity in mental health treatment; participating in, and sponsoring, community events; and so forth. In this day and age, giving lip service to issues of diversity seems to be somewhat trendy. A facility that truly honors cultural diversity reflects this in many ways, not just for the benefit of the clients, but also for the benefit of the staff.

5. *Does the facility make an effort to understand the needs of the community it serves?* Whom does the facility serve? What does the facility know about the community in which it is located? How does the facility assess the needs of the community, and how does it assess whether or not those needs are being met? The answer to this general question is perhaps the most important, for, if the facility does not make an effort to understand the community that it serves, few peo-ple's needs are likely to be met.

Addressing Barriers to Culturally Appropriate Treatment at the Individual Level

Providing culturally appropriate mental health services is not just the responsibility of the facility, but is a responsibility for each individual mental health care worker. Just as there are questions that hospitals and clinics can answer, there are several questions that clinicians can ask themselves when assessing their level of cultural sensitivity and understanding of their Asian American clients.

1. *Are you aware of how culture may influence the client's behaviors when interacting with you?* Culturally appropriate behaviors among Asian Americans may sometimes be mistakenly pathologized. For example, in many Asian cultures, deference to authority and cooperation are highly valued. Thus, it is not uncommon for many Asian American clients to avoid eye contact and to answer questions either very briefly or indirectly. These types of behaviors should neither be pathologized nor be a focus of treatment. The clinician must be patient and thorough when conducting assessments.

2. *How does the client understand his or her symptoms?* Kleinman (1977) suggested that, although the experience of illness symptoms might be universal, interpretation of those symptoms is culturally bound. He referred to this as the client's explanatory model of illness (EMI). That is, each of us may experience the same thing physically, but the meaning and source we attribute those symptoms to may be very different. Kleinman, Eisenberg, and Good (1978) further argued that, in order to improve treatment compliance, we need to deliver health care services in a manner congruent to the patient's EMIs, and not our own. If the treatment matches the patient's EMI, the patient will be more likely to comply, and hence feel better sooner.

3. *Are you respectful of the client?* Showing respect is particularly important for elderly Asian Americans. As indicated earlier in this chapter, elderly Asian Americans are viewed as wise and treated with reverence. Clinicians should consider their tone of voice and their manner of speech with such individuals. Explain what you are doing with the client and why you are doing it.

4. *Do you assess somatization and psychological distress separately?* In assessing symptoms, the clinician should attempt to differentiate between somatization and other psychological distress. If the client is experiencing somatic complaints, what is the etiology of those complaints? As Kleinman (1977) indicated, the actual source may be less important than the *perceived* source in implementing treatment.

5. *Do you assess depression and anxiety separately?* In general, differentiating between anxiety and depression is a difficult task for clinicians. This may be even more challenging for the clinician working with Asian Americans. Some Asian Americans may not use the same descriptors or terminology that non-Asian American clients will use in describing their symptoms. Thus, the clinician should ask for examples

and clarification from the client in attempting to differentiate between the two disorders. Clinicians should also be flexible and not interpret Western diagnostic categories rigidly. For example, an Asian American client might say that she has a "heavy heart" or a "troubled mind" instead of saying she is sad or is having difficulty concentrating and making decisions. A clinician who is not sensitive to cultural variation in symptom descriptions might actually misdiagnose someone and implement inappropriate treatment recommendations.

6. *Do you assess the role of drug and alcohol use on symptoms?* Although many clinicians believe that alcohol and drug use among Asian Americans is low, assessment of drug and alcohol use should be conducted with Asian American clients just as with any other client. Use of drugs or alcohol may affect an individual's attempt to cope with anxiety symptoms or may be the source of them.

7. *Do you assess the impact of symptoms on interpersonal relationships?* As interpersonal harmony is a valued aspect of many Asian Americans' lives, assessing the interpersonal relationships of Asian American clients might also assist the clinician in determining the presence of anxiety symptoms. Often, an individual might not be able to articulate specific psychological symptoms, but will be able to tell the clinician if he or she is experiencing impairment in relationships with loved ones and coworkers. In addition to self-report, the clinician may be able to obtain this information from the client's loved ones.

8. *Do you apply norms developed on European Americans to Asian Americans?* As there are few assessment tools developed specifically for Asian Americans, one might resort to using measures that have been developed and standardized on European Americans. Using norms from such measures to interpret and understand the psychological distress of an Asian American client may not only be culturally inappropriate, but may lead the clinician to make culturally incompatible treatment recommendations. As discussed earlier, it is hypothesized that getting a sense of how the *client* interprets his or her symptoms would be more beneficial for developing treatment interventions that the client will accept. Thus, although the clinician might use a measure standardized on an ethnically and culturally different group to get a sense of symptoms from a Western perspective, he or she needs to determine how helpful that information will be in the provision of effective treatment for the Asian American client.

9. *Do you assess the individual's socioeconomic status, social support, and employment status?* As with any other client, the clinician's awareness of the Asian American client's socioeconomic status, social support network, and employment status will give the clinician important information on the resources available to the client. Obviously, a client who is

employed, living above the poverty level, and has an extended social support network will have more resources for coping than would an individual who is not working, lives below the poverty level, and has few close friends and family members. For those Asian American clients who are employed, it would be important for the clinician to understand how many hours the client works per day, as well as how many jobs the individual has. It is highly likely that an immigrant Asian American is working more than 8 hours per day, or holding more than one job, in order to make ends meet. It is also possible that the individual is supporting a large number of family members, such as aunts, uncles, and cousins, in addition to his or her own immediate family.

10. *Are you aware of possible ethnic group differences in the expression of symptoms?* The emphasis here is to be aware of one's own stereotypes about Asian Americans. From reviewing the earlier section on within- and between-group differences among Asian Americans, as well as the section on culture-specific disorders, hopefully the reader is now aware that not all Asian Americans are the same, nor will they present in exactly the same manner with the same set of symptoms of a particular disorder. Clinicians must be adept at recognizing their own perceptions about people and how these might influence their expectations of Asian American clients.

11. *Are you aware of how ethnicity might affect the reporting of the severity of symptoms?* Research has indicated that many Asian Americans do not enter the mental health system until their distress is at a severe level. Given this, it is important for clinicians not to minimize the severity of symptoms should an Asian American self-present for treatment. Because the individual might feel somewhat uncomfortable about seeking mental health services, he or she might tend to minimize the extent of symptoms. That is why it is imperative for the clinician to assess how the symptoms are interfering with other areas in the client's life such as interpersonal relationships, as well as assessing the severity of symptoms themselves. For instance, it would be important to inquire about the extent to which the individual suffers from sleep and appetite disturbance, as well as how much of the time the individual spends worrying or engaging in compulsive behaviors, instead of simply asking if the person is experiencing those problems. The clinician must be sure to assess the severity of all of the relevant symptoms before making an assumption about the severity of distress.

12. *Do you assess how the environment might be maintaining and reinforcing anxiety symptoms?* Any behavioral therapist can explain that many inappropriate behaviors occur because they are reinforced by the individual's environment. Tanaka-Matsumi et al. (1996) suggest a comprehensive assessment of the individual's environment, which helps to

identify the aspects of the environment that may be exacerbating the anxiety symptoms. For example, a person may feel pressured and worried about work because of an overbearing supervisor. This, in conjunction with a significant other who may also be reinforcing the supervisor's unrealistic demands while the client is at home, may serve to reinforce the client's anxiety symptoms.

13. *Are you aware of how immigration experiences might relate to anxiety symptoms?* In working with Asian American immigrants, clinicians must be sensitive to how those experiences may have precipitated anxiety symptoms and, as discussed above, how the individual's current environment may be reinforcing those symptoms. Again, it is important to assess the level of trauma and difficulty of the individual's immigration experience, as well as the individual's current experiences with adapting to a new environment. This may best be conducted by asking the client to tell his or her story about coming to the United States, and asking for further elaboration when necessary, instead of asking the client numerous close-ended questions.

14. *Do you utilize the patient's social support network to support and maintain treatment compliance?* Because of the strong emphasis on family and community, the clinician may have numerous extratherapy resources at his or her disposal. If the client gives consent, family members, community or religious leaders, or family friends can be used as allies in the development and implementation of interventions outside of therapy. This automatically builds in a social support component, which will increase the likelihood of maintaining any gains made during treatment. The therapist may be surprised to find that a client is more likely to follow through with a suggestion made by a family member or friend, than if that same suggestion came from the therapist. An example of this is illustrated by S. Sue and Zane's (1987) work with a Chinese American woman. They successfully utilized the client's uncle as an intermediary in resolving a conflict between the client and her mother-in-law.

15. *Are you aware of the difficulties in using translation?* Many health care workers, particularly in urban settings, rely on translators when working with non-English-speaking clients. Extreme caution must be used, and the identity of the translator must be carefully considered. Use of a translator has a major impact on the reporting of symptoms, on family roles, and on how the client is treated by the health care worker. Clinicians cannot assume that they are getting an accurate interpretation of what the client is experiencing, and may actually be decreasing the likelihood of treatment compliance if the experience of translation is not a positive one for the client. Role reversal for example, a grandchild given more credibility than the grandparent who is the client—is a prime

example of how translation could be detrimental to the client. This is particularly evident in situations where the client is almost completely ignored by the clinician, who only speaks to the translator, rather than directly to the client. This kind of clinician behavior is in direct opposition to Asian cultural values of respect for older adults.

16. *Do you emphasize the goals of treatment and how treatment will lead to the goal?* S. Sue and Zane (1987) discuss how the client must have a sense of getting something out of treatment. They refer to this as "giving" on the part of the therapist, which in turns "buys" the therapist credibility. One of the most effective ways to do this with Asian American clients is to emphasize the goals of treatment and specifically, how the suggested treatment interventions will help the client to obtain those goals. In other words, it is important to emphasize that treatment is specific and time limited.

17. *Do you ask questions and seek consultation when you do not know something?* A final suggestion is not to be afraid to ask questions when feeling ignorant. Consulting with colleagues who have expertise in working with Asian Americans, reading articles and chapters such as this one, attending workshops, and, of course, asking the client questions directly are not only appropriate, but imperative. It is those therapists who are the *least* comfortable dealing with issues of ethnicity who likely need the *most* assistance in their work with Asian Americans. Often, clinicians forget that the richest resource on issues of ethnicity is their own clients.

In summary, this chapter reviewed some of the similarities and differences among the various Asian American ethnic groups. A brief review of the empirical research on anxiety disorders and Asian Americans was provided, as were suggestions for providing effective treatment for Asian Americans at both the institutional and individual level. The reader is encouraged to consult the references indicated in the chapter for more in-depth information on Asian Americans.

REFERENCES

Abueg, F. R., & Chun, K. M. (1996). Traumatization stress among Asians and Asian Americans. In A. J. Marsella, M. J. Friedman, E. T. Gerrity, & R. S. Scurfield (Eds.), *Ethnocultural aspects of posttraumatic stress disorder: Issues, research, and clinical applications.* Washington, DC: American Psychological Association.

Almirol, E. B. (1990). The economic adaptation of Filipino Americans in California. In S. Chan (Ed.), *Income and status differences between white and minority Americans.* Lewiston, NY: Edwin Mellen Press.

American Psychiatric Association. (1994). *Diagnostic and statistical manual of mental disorders* (4th ed.). Washington, DC: Author.

Anderson, J. N. (1983). Health and illness in Filipino immigrants. *Western Journal of Medicine, 139,* 811–819.

Aylesworth, L. S., Ossorio, P. G., & Osaki, L. T. (1980). Stress and mental health among Vietnamese in the United States. In R. Endo, S. Sue, & N. Wagner (Eds.), *Asian Americans: Social and psychological perspectives.* Palo Alto, CA: Science and Behavior Books.

Beiser, M., & Fleming, J. A. E. (1986). Measuring psychiatric disorder among Southeast Asian refugees. *Psychological Medicine, 16,* 627–639.

Bradshaw, C. K. (1994). Asian and Asian American women: Historical and political considerations in psychotherapy. In L. Comas-Díaz & B. Greene (Eds.), *Women of color: Integrating ethnic and gender identities in psychotherapy.* New York: Guilford Press.

Brown, T. R., Stein, K. M., Huang, K., & Harris, D. E. (1973). Mental illness and the role of mental health facilities in Chinatown. In S. Sue & N. Wagner (Eds.), *Asian Americans: Psychological perspectives.* Palo Alto, CA: Science and Behavior Books.

Cabezas, A., Shinagawa, L. H., & Kawaguchi, G. (1990). Income differentials between Asian Americans and White Americans in California, 1980. In S. Chan (Ed.), *Income and status differences between white and minority Americans.* Lewiston, NY: Edwin Mellen Press.

Chan, S. (1991). *Asian Americans: An interpretive history.* Boston: Twayne.

Cheung, F. K. (1991). The use of mental health services by ethnic minorities. In H. F. Myers, P. Wohlford, L. P. Guzman, & R. J. Echemendia (Eds.), *Ethnic minority perspectives on clinical training and services in psychology.* Washington, DC: American Psychological Association.

Chew, C. A., & Ogi, D. C. (1987). Asian American college student perspectives. *New Directions for Student Services, 38,* 39–48.

Chia, R. (1989). Pilot study: Family values of American versus Chinese-American parents. *Journal of the Asian American Psychological Association, 13,* 8–11.

Chin, J. L. (1983). Diagnostic considerations in working with Asian Americans. *American Journal of Orthopsychiatry, 53,* 100–109.

Choy, B. Y. (1979). *Koreans in America.* Chicago: Nelson-Hall.

Durvasula, R., & Sue, S. (1996). Severity of disturbance among Asian American outpatients. *Cultural Diversity and Mental Health, 2,* 43–51.

Felsman, J. K., Leong, F. T. L., Johnson, M. C., & Felsman, I. C. (1990). Estimates of psychological distress among Vietnamese refugees: Adolescents, unaccompanied minors and young adults. *Social Science and Medicine, 31,* 1251–1256.

Flaskerud, J. H., & Akutsu, P. D. (1993). Significant influence of participation in ethnic-specific programs on clinical diagnosis for Asian Americans. *Psychological Reports, 72,* 1228–1230.

Flaskerud, J. H., & Hu, L. (1992). Relationship of ethnicity to psychiatric diagnosis. *Journal of Nervous and Mental Disease, 180,* 296–303.

Fort, J. G., Watts, J. C., & Lesser, G. S. (1969). Cultural background and learning in young children. *Phi Delta Kappan, 50,* 386–388.

Fukuyama, M., & Greenfield, T. K. (1983). Dimensions of assertiveness in an Asian American student population. *Journal of Counseling Psychology, 30,* 429–432.

Hess, R. D., Chang, C., & McDevitt, T. M. (1987). Cultural variations in family beliefs about children's performance in mathematics: Comparisons among People's Republic of China, Chinese-American, and Caucasian-American families. *Journal of Educational Psychology, 79,* 179–188.

Hinton, W. L., Chen, Y. J., Du, N., Tran, C. G., Lu, F. G., Miranda, J., & Faust, S. (1993). DSM-III-R disorders in Vietnamese refugees: Prevalence and correlates. *Journal of Nervous and Mental Disease, 181,* 113–122.

Ho, C. K. (1990). An analysis of domestic violence in Asian American communities: A multicultural approach to counseling. *Women and Therapy, 9,* 129–150.

Hsu, F. L. K. (1971). Psychosocial homeostasis and Jen: Conceptual tools for advancing psychological anthropology. *American Anthropologist, 73,* 23–44.

Hsu, J., Tseng, W., Ashton, G., McDermott, J., & Char, W. (1985). Family interaction patterns among Japanese-American and Caucasian families in Hawaii. *American Journal of Psychiatry, 142,* 577–581.

Hurh, W. M., & Kim, K. C. (1984). *Korean immigrants in America.* Cranbury, NJ: Associated University Press.

Imada, H. (1989). Cross-language comparisons of emotional terms with special reference to the concept of anxiety. *Japanese Psychological Research, 31,* 10–19.

Iwamasa, G. Y. (1996). Acculturation of Asian American university students. *Assessment, 3,* 99–102.

Johnson, F. A., Marsella, A. J., & Johnson, C. L. (1974). Social and psychological aspects of verbal behavior in Japanese-Americans. *American Journal of Psychiatry, 131,* 580–583.

Kalish, R., & Moriwaki, S. (1973). The world of the elderly Asian American. *Journal of Social Issues, 29,* 187–209.

Kim, B. L. C. (1980). *Korean American child at school and at home.* Technical report to the Administration for Children, Youth, and Families. Washington, DC: U.S. Department of Health, Education and Welfare.

Kim-Goh, M. (1993). Conceptualization of mental illness among Korean-American clergymen and implications for mental health service delivery. *Community Mental Health Journal, 29,* 405–412.

Kinzie, D. J., & Tseng, W. (1978). Cultural aspects of psychiatric clinic utilization: A cross-cultural study in Hawaii. *International Journal of Social Psychiatry, 24,* 177–188.

Kirmayer, L. J. (1991). The place of culture in psychiatric nosology: Taijin Kyofusho and DSM-III-R. *Journal of Nervous and Mental Disease, 179,* 19–28.

Kitano, H. H. L., & Kikumura, A. (1976). The Japanese American family. In C. H. Mindel & R. W. Habenstein (Eds.), *Ethnic families in America.* New York: Elsevier.

Kleinknecht, R. A., Dinnel, D. L., Tanouye-Wilson, S., & Lonner, W. J. (1994). Cultural variation in social anxiety and phobia: A study of *Taijin Kyofusho. Behavior Therapist, 17,* 175–178.

Kleinman, A. M. (1977). Depression, somatization, and the "new cross-cultural psychiatry." *Social Science and Medicine, 11,* 3–10.

Kleinman, A. M., Eisenberg, L., & Good, B. (1978). Culture, illness and care: Clinical lessons from anthropological and cross-cultural research. *Annals of Internal Medicine, 88,* 251–288.

Kroll, J., Habenicht, M., Mackenzie, T., Yang, M., Chan, S., Vang, T., Nguyen, T., Ly, M., Phommasouvanh, B., Nguyen, H., Vang, Y., Souvannasoth, L., & Caugao, R. (1989). Depression and posttraumatic stress disorder in Southeast Asian refugees. *American Journal of Psychiatry, 146,* 1592–1597.

Lee, J., & Cynn, V. (1991). Issues in counseling 1. 5 generation Korean Americans. In C. Lee & B. Richardson (Eds.), *Multicultural issues in counseling: New approaches to diversity.* Alexandria, VA: American Association for Counseling and Development.

Lin, C., & Fu, V. (1990). A comparison of child-rearing practices among Chinese, immigrant Chinese, and Caucasian-American parents. *Child Development, 61,* 429–433.

Lin, K. (1983). *Hwa-Byung*: A Korean culture-bound syndrome? *American Journal of Psychiatry, 140,* 105–107.

Lin, K., Inui, T. S., Kleinman, A. M., & Womack, W. M. (1982). Sociocultural determinants of the help-seeking behavior of patients with mental illness. *Journal of Nervous and Mental Disease, 170,* 78–85.

Lin, K., Lau, J. K. C., Yamamoto, J., Zheng, Y., Kim, H., Cho, K., & Nakasaki, G. (1992). *Hwa Byung*: A community study of Korean Americans. *Journal of Nervous and Mental Disease, 180,* 386–391.

Lin, N., Ensel, W. M., Simeone, R. S., & Kuo, W. (1979). Social support, stressful life events, and illness: A model and empirical test. *Journal of Health and Social Behavior, 20,* 108–119.

Lyman, S. M. (1974). *Chinese Americans.* New York: Random House.

McDermott, J. F., Char, W., Robillard, A., Hsu, J., Tseng, W., & Ashton, G. (1984). Cultural variations in family attitudes and their implications for therapy. In S. Chess & A. Thomas (Eds.), *Annual progress in child psychiatry and child development.* New York: Brunner/Mazel.

Miller, M. D., Reynolds, R. A., & Cambra, R. E. (1987). The influence of gender and culture on language intensity. *Communication Monographs, 54,* 101–105.

Mollica, R. F., Wyshak, G., de Marneffe, D., Khuon, F., & Lavelle, J. (1987). Indochinese versions of the Hopkins Symptom Checklist-25: A screening instrument for the psychiatric care of refugees. *American Journal of Psychiatry, 144,* 497–500.

Morales, R. F. (1974). *Makibaca: The Filipino American struggle.* Darby, MT: Mountain View.

Nagata, D. (1989). Long-term effects of the Japanese American internment camps: Impact upon the children of the internees. *Journal of the Asian American Psychological Association, 13,* 48–55.

Payton, C. (1985). Addressing the special needs of minority women. *New Directions for Student Services, 29,* 75–90.

Petersen, W. (1978). Chinese Americans and Japanese Americans. In T. Sowell (Ed.), *Essays and data on American ethnic groups.* Washington, DC: Urban Institute.

Phinney, J. (1990). Ethnic identity in adolescents and adults: Review of research. *Psychological Bulletin, 108,* 499–514.

Shibutani, T., & Kwan, K. (1965). *Ethnic stratification: A comparative approach.* London: MacMillan.

Shon, S., & Ja, D. (1982). Asian families. In M. McGoldrick, J. K. Pearce, & J. Giordano (Eds.), *Ethnicity and family therapy.* New York: Guilford Press.

Shu, R., & Satele, A. S. (1977). *The Samoan community in Southern California: Conditions and needs.* Chicago: Asian American Mental Health Research Center.

Smither, R., & Rodriguez-Giegling, M. (1979). Marginality, modernity, and anxiety in Indochinese refugees. *Journal of Cross-Cultural Psychology, 10,* 469–478.

Sollenberger, R. T. (1968). Chinese American child-rearing practices and juvenile delinquency. *Journal of Social Psychology, 74,* 13–23.

Strom, R., Park, S. H., & Daniels, S. (1987). Child rearing dilemmas of Korean immigrants to the United States. *International Journal of Experimental Research in Education, 24,* 91–102.

Sue, D., Ino, S., & Sue, D. (1983). Nonassertiveness of Asian Americans: An inaccurate assumption? *Journal of Counseling Psychology, 30,* 581–588.

Sue, D., Sue, D. M., & Ino, S. (1990). Assertiveness and social anxiety in Chinese-American women. *Journal of Psychology, 124,* 155–163.

Sue, D. W. (1989). Ethnic identity: The impact of two cultures on the psychological development of Asians in America. In D. R. Atkinson, G. Morten, & D. W. Sue (Eds.), *Counseling American minorities: A cross-cultural perspective.* Dubuque, IA: WC Brown.

Sue, S., & McKinney, H. (1975). Asian Americans in the community health care system. *American Journal of Orthopsychiatry, 45,* 111–118.

Sue, S., & Morishima, J. K. (1982). *The mental health of Asian Americans.* San Francisco: Jossey-Bass.

Sue, S., & Sue, D. W. (1973). Chinese-American personality and mental health. In S. Sue & N. Wagner (Eds.), *Asian Americans: Psychological perspectives.* Palo Alto, CA: Science and Behavior Books.

Sue, S., & Zane, N. (1987). The role of culture and cultural techniques in psychotherapy: A critique and reformulation. *American Psychologist, 42,* 37–45.

Suinn, R. M., Rickland-Figueroa, K., Lew, S., & Vigil, P. (1987). The Suinn–Lew Asian Self-Identity Acculturation Scale: An initial report. *Educational and Psychological Measurement, 47,* 401–407.

Takeuchi, D. T., Kuo, H., Kim, K., & Leaf, P. J. (1989). Psychiatric symptom dimensions among Asian Americans and Native Hawaiians: An analysis of the Symptom Checklist. *Journal of Community Psychology, 17,* 319–329.

Tanaka-Matsumi, J., Seiden, D. Y., & Lam, K. N. (1996). Cross-cultural functional analysis: A strategy for culturally informed clinical assessment. *Cognitive and Behavioral Practice, 3,* 215–234.

Tien, L. (1994). Southeast Asian American refugee women. In L. Comas-Díaz & B. Greene (Eds.), *Women of color: Integrating ethnic and gender identities in psychotherapy.* New York: Guilford Press.

Tran, T. V. (1993). Psychological traumas and depression in a sample of Vietnamese people in the United States. *Health and Social Work, 18,* 184–194.

Tseng, W., Asai, M., Kitanishi, K., McLaughlin, D. G., & Kyomen, H. (1992). Diagnostic patterns of social phobia: Comparison in Tokyo and Hawaii. *Journal of Nervous and Mental Disease, 180,* 380–385.

Tsui, P., & Schultz, G. (1988). Ethnic factors in group process: Cultural dynamics in multi-ethnic therapy groups. *American Journal of Orthopsychiatry, 58,* 378–384.

Uba, L. (1994). *Asian Americans: Personality patterns, identity, and mental health.* New York: Guilford Press.

U. S. Bureau of the Census. (1992). *Census of population and housing* (Summary Tape file 3A, 1990 [CD90-3A] [CD-ROM]). Washington, DC: Author.

U. S. Department of Health and Human Services, Public Health Service, Health Care Financing Administration, U. S. G. P. O. (1991). *International Classification of Diseases, Ninth revision, Clinical modification.* Washington, DC: Author.

Westermeyer, J., Neider, J., & Vang, T. F. (1984). Acculturation and mental health: A study of Hmong Refugees at 1. 5 and 3. 5 years postmigration. *Social Science and Medicine, 18,* 87–91.

Yang, J. (1991). Career counseling of Chinese American women: Are they in limbo? *Career Development Quarterly, 39,* 350–359.

Yao, E. (1985). A comparison of family characteristics of Asian-American and Anglo-American high achievers. *International Journal of Comparative Sociology, 26,* 198–208.

Yi, K., Zane, N., & Sue, S. (1986). Cognitive appraisal of assertion responses among Asian and Caucasian Americans. *Asian American Psychological Association Journal, 13,* 65–68.

Young, N. (1972). Changes in values and strategies among Chinese in Hawaii. *Sociology and Social Research, 26,* 228–241.

Yu, K., & Kim, L. (1983). The growth and development of Korean-American children. In G. Powell (Ed.), *The psychosocial development of minority group children.* New York: Brunner/Mazel.

Zane, N., & Sue, S. (1991). Culturally responsive mental health services for Asian Americans: Treatment and training issues. In H. F. Myers, P. Wohlford, L. P. Guzman, & R. J. Echemendia (Eds.), *Ethnic minority perspectives on clinical training and services in psychology.* Washington, DC: American Psychological Association.

Zane, N., Sue, S., Hu, L., & Kwon, J. (1991). Asian American assertion: A social learning analysis of cultural differences. *Journal of Counseling Psychology, 38,* 63–70.

7

~~~

Orthodox Jews

CHERYL M. PARADIS
STEVEN FRIEDMAN
MARJORIE L. HATCH
ROBERT ACKERMAN

A consensus has evolved in recent years that supports the conclusion that successful treatment must incorporate an understanding of the client's cultural beliefs (Gaw, 1993; Jenkins, 1994). This approach has been reflected in the modifications of the fourth edition of the *Diagnostic and Statistical Manual of Mental Disorders* (DSM-IV), which include a lengthy addendum on "Culture and Psychiatric Diagnosis" edited by the steering committee, National Institute of Mental Health Group on Culture and Diagnosis (American Psychiatric Association, 1994). Much of the literature on psychotherapy with Jewish clients concerns either psychoanalytic treatment of non-Orthodox, assimilated Jews (Jucovy, 1992) or the psychological effects of the Holocaust on its survivors and their offspring (Davidson, 1980). Little has been published, however, concerning the treatment of anxiety disorders in Orthodox Jews. Many of the concerns of Orthodox Jews, as people who define themselves in terms of their religion, are similar to those of other religious groups including Muslims, Mormons, and Seventh Day Adventists. Therefore, many of the issues we discuss may have utility for other religious groups. It is important that mental health professionals understand and appreciate the cultural values and norms (mores) of the Orthodox Jewish community so as to provide effective treatment. Although little research has been done on the use of cognitive-behavioral treatment in treating anxiety disorders in a possible wide range of religious groups, the importance of providing culturally sensitive treatment has been addressed (Hayes & Toarmino, 1995; Greenberg & Witztum, 1989; Suess & Halpern, 1989).

Providing psychological treatment to Orthodox Jews requires that any therapeutic approach incorporate this group's specific religious beliefs, societal values, and norms. In this paper we review some cultural issues and how they impact on the treatment of anxiety disorders in Orthodox Jews.

Orthodox Jews share the core belief that the Torah (see Table 7.1 for glossary of terms) and the laws of God are nonnegotiable and unchangeable. They live in close-knit communities and hold values emphasizing family and community. It is important for the therapist to be aware of the laws and customs concerning everyday behavior, the distinct roles of men and women, and observance of holidays and the Sabbath. This awareness is necessary both in developing a therapeutic alliance as well as designing a successful treatment approach. In our clinical experience, Orthodox Jews usually seek treatment only when the anxiety symptoms severely interfere with functioning. The stigma concerning mental illness affects the choice of a therapist, *in vivo* work, and participation in support groups. Our experience is that cognitive-behavioral treatment can be quite successful when the patients' values are respected and incorporated into the treatment process. Consultation and collaboration with a rabbi often aids in treatment, and we will discuss this issue at a later point.

Our Anxiety Disorders clinic is located in Brooklyn, New York, an area of great cultural and religious diversity. We have been afforded the opportunity to treat clients with anxiety disorders from a wide spectrum of cultural groups (Friedman, Paradis, & Hatch, 1994; Friedman, Hatch, Paradis, Popkin, & Shalita, 1993) including various Orthodox Jewish groups. Judaism has three major subgroups: Orthodox, Conservative, and Reform. Although this chapter will focus specifically on the treatment of Orthodox Jews, many of the issues discussed may also be relevant in the treatment of non-Orthodox Jews. We will provide an overview of the Orthodox Jewish Community and how certain issues, such as views of mental illness, confidentiality, family relationships, and religious holidays and rituals, impact on the therapeutic process and alliance.

TABLE 7.1. Glossary of Terms

Chumrah:	An acceptable, stringent religiosity.
Halakah:	Jewish law comprised of written and oral traditions.
Hasidism:	Religious movement founded in the first half of the 18th century in Eastern Europe. In opposition to rationalism, it emphasized the individual's closeness to God and ties to a charismatic leader (*rebbe*). Major sects continue, often in direct descent from the original founder.
Holocaust:	The organized mass persecution and annihilation of European Jewry by the Nazis (1933–1945).
Kashruth:	Jewish dietary laws (e.g., meat and dairy are never mixed, no pork or shellfish, etc.)
Kosher:	Ritually permitted food.
Mitzvah:	A commandment to perform certain deeds. Also used to refer to a good or charitable deed.
Niddah:	A woman during the period of menstruation and 7 days after cessation when no physical contact between husband and wife is permitted.
Reb, rebbe:	Yiddish form for rabbi, applied generally to a teacher or a Hasidic rabbi.
Synagogue:	Place of worship, the center of religious and social life for Orthodox Jews.
Talmud:	"Teaching,," the authoritative body of Jewish law and tradition codified in the 3rd–5th centuries comprising both *Halakah* and *Aggadah* ("folklore").
Torah:	Scroll containing the first five books of the Bible for reading in the synagogue. Also can refer to the entire body of traditional Jewish teaching.
Yeshiva:	An academy devoted to the study of religious and rabbinical literature. In the Orthodox Jewish tradition sexes are educated separately. Currently, in these schools, children receive both religious and secular education.

BRIEF OVERVIEW OF THE ORTHODOX JEWISH COMMUNITY

There are approximately 14 million Jews worldwide, with over 5 million residing in the United States (*Academic American Encyclopedia*, 1993), and there are approximately 250,000 adult Jews living in Brooklyn, one third of whom define themselves as Orthodox (Horowitz, 1993). Subgroups of the Orthodox Jewish community vary in the strictness of their interpretation of the *Halakah* (Jewish law composed of written and oral traditions) and differ somewhat in their cultural and familial traditions. These differences are generally related to the country of origin of the patient or their parents. The core set of beliefs shared by all Orthodox Jews is the strict interpretation of the Torah (five books they believe were given directly to Moses by God) (Hirsch, 1967). The Torah and its laws are interpreted in written commentaries including the *Talmud*. Although applications of the Torah may vary in different circumstances and settings, its laws are viewed as unchangeable and nonnegotiable. The laws govern each individual's relationship with God and his or her relationships with others. There are specific prescriptions for every aspect of life including, but not limited to, laws governing marriage, divorce, family relationships, sexual behavior, charity, and observance of the Sabbath and holidays, as well as the laws of *kashruth* (dietary prohibitions and practices for animal slaughter and food preparation).

There are 613 *mitzvoth* (commandments, laws) taken from the Torah that prescribe or proscribe behavior. Although some groups of Orthodox Jews are more "modern" in that they may be more assimilated into modern American culture in their appearance and values, the spectrum also includes many groups of Hasidim. These include the Lubavitch and Satmar Hasidic sects, which continue the traditions of 18th- and 19th-century Europe in their dress and language (often speaking Yiddish). Hasidic groups originate from Central and Eastern Europe and follow a particular dynasty of rabbinical leaders. There may be significant differences in social behavior among the Hasidic sects. Many Lubavitch Hasidim, for example, expressed the belief that their rabbi was the Messiah as prophesied in the Torah. The Satmar Hasidim believe that the State of Israel should not exist until brought about by the arrival of the Messiah and some Hasidim campaign against the existence of Israel as a modern state.

However, Orthodox Jews will generally share important religious and cultural values that sharply differ from those of the modern secular world emphasizing individuality and autonomy (Hirsch, 1967). Most importantly, Orthodox Jews define themselves primarily as members of a community. They often strive to separate themselves and their community from mainstream society in order to maintain their traditional way of life and adherence to their religious values, beliefs, and behaviors.

Jewish law forbids traveling in cars on the Sabbath and holidays; therefore, Orthodox Jews need to live within walking distance of their synagogue. This requirement promotes a closeness in the community and favors locating the community in an urban setting. Members of Orthodox Jewish communities usually live near each other in close-knit, small communities.

Holidays and the weekly Sabbath set the pace and structure of Orthodox Jewish life. Holidays are both solemn and joyful and may also consist of major or minor fast days. Time and rituals are orchestrated in a schedule of observance and are adhered to without deviation. It is important for the therapist to become knowledgeable about these events in order to conduct treatment effectively. A listing of major holidays is included in (Table 7.2).

TABLE 7.2. Jewish Holidays and Fasts

Name	Date	Significance
Hanukkah	December	An 8-day holiday to honor the victory over the Hellenic Syrians, the rededication of the Temple in 165 B.C.E., and various miracles.
Purim	February or March	A joyous festival to celebrate the defeat of the Persian Haman in the 5th century B.C.E.
Rosh Hashanah	September or October	A 2-day holiday. The Jewish New Year that begins the 10 Days of Repentance and culminates in Yom Kippur.
Sabbath (Shabbat)	Weekly	A day of rest, prayer, and study, beginning at sundown on Friday and ending an hour after sundown on Saturday.
Simhath Torah	September or October	A day of rejoicing in the completion of the reading of the Torah.
Shavuoth	May or June	A 2-day holiday. The Feast of Weeks to celebrate receiving the Torah at Mount Sinai.
Succoth (Feast of Tabernacles)	September or October	A harvest festival that recreates the huts that Jews built and lived in, symbolizing the 40 years Jews wandered in the wilderness after exodus from Egypt prior to entering the Promised Land.
Tishah B'Ab	July or August	A fast day to mourn the destruction of the First Temple in 586 B.C.E. and the Second Temple in 70 A.D.
Tu B'Shebat	January or February	Arbor Day to celebrate the planting of trees in Israel.
Yom Kippur	September or October	The Day of Atonement, the holiest day in the Jewish Year. A fast day.
Passover	March or April	A Festival of Freedom to commemorate the exodus from Egypt.

Note. The Jewish calendar is a lunar calendar. The beginning of a Jewish day starts at sunset and ends at sunset, 25 hours later.

VIEW OF MENTAL ILLNESS

Orthodox Jews often view mental illness as a disease that needs to be concealed. As in other ethnic religious groups, when individuals begin to suffer anxiety symptoms they first look for help from immediate family or religious leaders (Neighbors, 1988). Orthodox individuals generally do not seek the help of a mental health professional until symptoms grossly interfere with functioning in the family or at work and school and after attempts to get help from the clergy or family have proved unsuccessful. The family and/or rabbinical leaders may actively discourage consulting a mental health professional. The family or a rabbinical leader may be concerned that the mental health professional would blame the patient's religious beliefs for the psychiatric symptoms or recommend a break with the religion or the community. At times, the rabbi may strongly encourage the patient to seek care from an Orthodox Jewish therapist. Interestingly, historically many Orthodox Jewish religious leaders preferred to refer a member to a non-Jewish therapist rather than a nonreligious, assimilated Jew, who was thought to have rejected the traditions of their people or to have negative attitudes or unresolved conflicts about their own Jewish background.

FAMILY RELATIONS

Family relationship issues of Orthodox Jews greatly impact the therapeutic process as is true in many family-oriented ethnic and religious groups. For example, for Orthodox Jews loyalty to family and traditions appears similar to the issues for Asian Americans discussed by Iwamasa (Chapter 6, this volume).

An important issue involves sex roles in the Orthodox Jewish community. The Torah provides a code of living that lays out different requirements for men and women (Hirsch, 1967). Women are primarily responsible for running the household, and men are primarily responsible for financial support and many religious obligations (obligation to study the Torah, certain prayers, etc.). Men are strongly encouraged to continue religious learning and study throughout their lives. The value of studying may supersede financial responsibilities, and it is common for a woman after marriage to work and support her husband's study of the Torah (wives actively encourage and support this pursuit of learning). Some couples continue this arrangement for many years, being financially supported by parents and other relatives.

Recent changes in American society have prompted women to work outside of the home as a means to provide additional income, establish autonomy, and enhance self-esteem. Although some Orthodox Jews support these goals, many do not. For example, women in some Hasidic sects are driven by male relatives or use car services because it is considered immodest for women to drive; similarly, the use of public transportation with the resulting mingling of sexes is avoided if possible. This does not mean that Orthodox women do not strive to achieve. Instead, opportunities can be found for Orthodox women to achieve within the community in defined roles by serving as volunteers in communal organizations such as *bikur cholim* (visiting the sick) or as teachers in the *yeshiva* (religious school). These realities and values need to be understood and respected by the therapist. The non-Orthodox therapist must be aware of any personal bias and adjust the treatment goals to meet the needs of each individual Orthodox client, which may differ significantly from those of non-Orthodox women (Ackerman, 1982). This issue is exemplified in the following case example.

> Ms. A., a 30-year-old Orthodox woman, came with her husband for treatment of her panic disorder and agoraphobia. Cognitive-behavioral treatment, combining relaxation training and exposure, was effective in decreasing the frequency of panic attacks. However, her continuing anxiety and depressive symptoms appeared related to poor self esteem because, in her view, she "did nothing important in her life."
>
> The therapist, who had relatively little experience working with Orthodox clients, naively encouraged her to explore career options. This intervention was met with much resistance from the client and her husband. It became clear that the couple's priority was for her to meet family demands (i.e., taking care of the children and household). Supervision from an Orthodox therapist suggested Ms. A. do volunteer work in the community. This was a more culturally appropriate intervention. This work helped her develop interpersonal skills and enhance self-esteem. The therapist was thus more effective in working with the client when she examined her own biases and values about women's roles vis-à-vis career and family.

It is also important that the therapist become knowledgeable concerning the many Jewish laws governing sexual behavior. The therapist, due to lack of knowledge of cultural mores, may recommend daily physical intimacy as a way to improve a marital relationship. The therapist needs to be aware of the laws of *taharat hamishpachah* ("family purity") including the laws of *niddah*. This law proscribes physical intimacy, even touching, from the start of menstruation until 7 days after the cessation of menstruation. Sexual activity can be resumed only after the woman has undergone ritual immersion in a *mikvah* (a body of water specifically utilized for this purpose). The therapist must respect these restrictions and promote intimacy through verbal communication during these times of physical separation (Ostrov, 1978).

As in other cultures, many Orthodox individuals may seek treatment for anxiety symptoms that were precipitated by marital conflict (Hafner, 1982). Treatment of non-Orthodox clients often involves examining the marital relationship, promoting greater individuation, or even encouraging separation or divorce. It is crucial for the non-Orthodox therapist to appreciate the sanctity of marriage within this community. As is true in other cultures, dissolution of a marriage is often not a viable option and only occurs in extreme situations of irreconcilable and continuous strife or physical abuse. Thus, the goal of treatment might be to improve the marital relationship and reduce the client's anxiety symptoms. Conflict can be addressed directly in marital counseling, and, although this is an acceptable treatment approach for many Orthodox clients, some clients with marital discord may resist a clinician's referral for marital counseling. Interestingly, when clients' anxiety symptoms improve with individual cognitive-behavioral treatment, they often report that their marriage is more satisfying or less conflictual. These issues are exemplified in the following case example.

Ms. B., a 41-year-old mother of four, was referred by her primary care physician (a member of the same Hasidic sect) for the treatment of severe panic attacks and spreading agoraphobia. Before making the referral, the physician asked to speak to us about our "treatment philosophy and approach." He reported that his patient had suffered from panic attacks for at least 10 years. However, her attacks, which were sporadic and interfered minimally with her functioning, had intensified over the past 2 years as a result of marital problems. The physician was familiar with the patient's history of school separation anxiety and a mother with lifelong and severe agoraphobia. The physician was also aware that the patient's husband wanted to be certain that the focus of treatment would be to help Ms. B. develop coping strategies. The physician knew the patient's husband and described him as "at times loving but at times a rigid and angry individual" who would not agree to couples counseling. The husband perceived his wife's panic symptoms as "her problems."

In an initial session, Ms. B. agreed that the stress of her conflictual marital relationship had contributed to a worsening of her symptoms, but she did not believe that couples treatment would result in any changes in her husband's behavior. She did not desire or expect that she would ever leave the relationship. She wanted help in "getting back to how I was, and making the best of it." Treatment consisted of a cognitive-behavioral approach. She was taught coping strategies to

deal with her fear of bodily sensations. A psychoeducational component and graduated exposure were effective in decreasing her anxiety
symptoms. Marital relationship issues were not directly addressed,
but, interestingly, the patient reported that as her anxiety symptoms
decreased, her relationship with her husband improved.

The community places great importance on the respect for parents
and elders, and this may affect treatment. The task of complete history
taking can be made more difficult because clients are often reluctant to
offer any information that may imply criticism of their parents. It is
important to avoid mistaking this reticence as uncooperativeness, or
denial when in fact it may be merely a reflection of a strongly held
cultural value (one of the Ten Commandments is to "honor your father
and mother"). Awareness of and sensitivity to this value are required
to encourage the client to discuss relevant family problems or history.
The law against *lashon hara* (literally translated as "evil speech" but
figuratively meaning gossip) further complicates the therapist's work
in taking a complete history. Clients may believe that giving a family
history violates this law, but at times they may also use it to avoid
facing or conveying conflictual material. This reluctance is seen in the
following case example.

> Mr. C., a 35-year-old Hasidic male, contacted the clinic because of
> severe panic attacks and agoraphobia. His ability to work and travel
> had become increasingly impaired over the previous 10 years. For
> many years, he avoided flying in planes, even for necessary business
> trips. Over the last year, his symptoms had worsened significantly to
> the point that he was unable to travel from Brooklyn to his office in
> Manhattan. When questioned about his understanding of the causes
> of his worsened agoraphobic symptoms, he was unable to offer an
> explanation and denied any recent family stressors. In the second
> session, which he attended with his wife, the therapist asked her view
> of why his long-standing, moderate problems had worsened so
> quickly. Very reluctantly his wife reported that "my husband's mother
> may be dying from breast cancer." Mr. C. had been reluctant to share
> this piece of information because he felt "it would be blaming, and
> be disrespectful to my mother." Mrs. C. stated she understood her
> husband's feelings and his decision to withhold information. Cogni-
> tive-behavioral treatment was effective in improving his functioning
> after the stressor of his mother's illness was identified and incorpo-
> rated into the treatment.
>   In this particular case, Mrs. C. was able to point out to her
> husband that his anxiety and panic symptoms would increase if he
> visited his mother or even if a sibling would call to talk about his

mother's health or treatment. Once this was pointed out, Mr. C. was able to understand the connection between "thoughts and feelings." At a certain point in treatment, a homework assignment was to provoke symptoms purposely by "increasing visits to his mother" and see that he could tolerate the anxiety without avoidance or fleeing.

The Torah states, "Be fruitful and multiply," and the Orthodox Jewish community places great value on having many children. Raising a large family, of course, can create stress and exacerbate a variety of anxiety disorders. A simplistic approach, however, of advising a client to limit family size can lead to an abrupt termination of treatment. Religious beliefs and the psychological urge to "replace" relatives murdered during the Holocaust support the practice of having large families. It is important that the goal of therapy be to help individuals cope with the stress of large and demanding families.

CONFIDENTIALITY

The importance of confidentiality for Orthodox Jews cannot be overly stressed. Their concerns regarding confidentiality, to the uninformed therapist, may appear to be almost "paranoid-like." Issues regarding confidentiality will affect an Orthodox Jew's choice of a psychotherapist and *in vivo* work. Clients who may be concerned about encountering an Orthodox therapist in a social or religious setting may choose to work with a therapist who is not an Orthodox Jew. This issue needs to be explored during the initial evaluation session.

Therapists working with clients with anxiety disorders often recommend that the individual talk with others about their symptoms, join support groups, and become less secretive about their disorder. These interventions are not generally used with Orthodox Jewish clients. Because members of the community are generally not educated about anxiety disorders, a patient's reputation can be adversely affected if his or her condition becomes known in the community.

The need to keep the anxiety disorder and treatment secret is great because of the widespread prejudice against those with mental illness in these close-knit communities. The term *"shanda"* is used to describe the shame of being "marked" by any secret (e.g., behaving in a callous manner, engaging in illegal or criminal activities, etc.). This *shanda* also includes mental retardation or mental illness in the family. Concern about one's reputation inhibits Orthodox Jews from discussing treatment with those outside the immediate family. Joining a support group or performing *in vivo* work in their neighborhood is generally not recommended. The therapist may recommend readings from Orthodox Jewish clinicians as useful adjuncts in therapy (Twersky, 1993). This literature, focused specifically for the Orthodox Jewish community, is helpful in destigmatizing anxiety disorders.

Orthodox Jewish clients may refuse to do *in vivo* work in their own neighborhood. They may be concerned that others who notice them with a nonreligious therapist may speculate about their relationship with an individual who is obviously not from the community. Clients who work with an Orthodox therapist may fear that the therapist will be recognized by others as a mental health professional. These realistic concerns need to be considered and discussed when designing *in vivo* exercises and in scheduling patients. Thus, a therapist should avoid scheduling consecutive office visits for patients of the same Orthodox community. A chance meeting might cause unnecessary shame and embarrassment.

As in other cultures, an Orthodox Jew with anxiety disorder may feel so ashamed of symptoms that he or she may avoid discussing the disorder even with a spouse. Nevertheless, our clinical experience with Orthodox Jews suggests that it is important and necessary to include spouses to some extent in the therapy process (Hafner, 1982; Friedman, 1987). However, this issue may need to be slowly and sensitively handled, as is shown in the following example.

Mr. D., a 26-year-old male, married for 2 years, contacted our clinic for treatment of his obsessions. He first experienced intrusive obsessions at the age of 16. At that time he engaged in compulsive cognitive activities to "neutralize" his bad thoughts. At first, his symptoms were relatively minor and interfered minimally with his intensive religious studies. However, his symptoms gradually worsened after his marriage.

On initial consultation he reported that he often stayed in the bathroom for nearly an hour so as to complete his rituals in privacy. The therapist recommended a joint session with his wife to discuss her view of the problem. He initially refused, because he had never told her of his symptoms and feared the shame and embarrassment he might feel or that his wife would leave him. It was gently pointed out that his compulsive rituals consumed many hours a day and that his wife probably realized something was wrong. He was reassured that sharing this secret with his wife would not necessarily put undue stress on him or their relationship, which he had described as an excellent one. Reluctantly, he agreed to her attending a joint session.

Mrs. D. reported that for years she had been aware of many of her husband's strange behaviors, including his lengthy trips to the bathroom and various writing and reading repetition rituals. She expressed relief on hearing that his symptoms were caused by an obsessive–compulsive disorder because she feared he had become psychotic or was on the verge of a complete nervous breakdown. Mr. D. responded well to individual and couples cognitive-behavioral treatment of his obsessive–compulsive (primarily exposure and response prevention).

In this case we had Mrs. D. help her husband keep the initial baseline record of his symptoms. In particular, Mr. D. was always intensively involved in religious studies and he was somewhat embarrassed by his poor ability to read and write English. As a cotherapist, Mrs. D. helped keep track of his symptoms as well as the amount of time he would expose himself to stimuli without engaging in rituals.

An Orthodox client's reluctance to discuss his or her anxiety disorder with others in the community may also impact decisions related to courtship and marriage. Members of Hasidic and other Orthodox communities begin dating for the sole purpose of selecting an appropriate marriage partner. The length of courtship varies among Orthodox groups, but an extended dating relationship of a year or more before the couple weds is not common. In the Hasidic community, a couple may decide that two to six dates is sufficient time for them to decide whether or not to marry and a "date" may actually consist of the young couple meeting "privately" for a brief period in the girl's home.

When an Orthodox Jew reaches a certain age, he or she begins the courtship process and takes on adult responsibilities. A young man may continue his studies and/or find productive employment. A young woman may continue to pursue educational or work-related skills; however, the primary goal is usually to "create a home and start a family." Individuals with a disabling physical or mental condition are often deemed not fit or ready to marry. They postpone the dating process until their conditions improve. Many Orthodox Jews with anxiety disorders have kept this secret from the extended community. Their symptoms are known only by immediate family members, which protects their reputation and chances for a good "match."

When an Orthodox Jewish individual starts to date, he or she is asserting to the community his or her fitness and readiness to marry. The decision to engage in courtship may pose a religious/ethical dilemma for individuals with moderate to severe anxiety disorders. Our approach is first to assess the extent of how their anxiety disorder interferes with functioning. Many individuals with anxiety disorders can fulfill their marital responsibilities. Their anxiety symptoms may only interfere with travel or participating in large social and religious gatherings. We suggest, as is advised by most rabbinical authorities, that our Orthodox Jewish clients not disclose details of their symptoms indiscriminately with those they date once or twice. Only when the couple begins seriously to consider marriage should the client disclose details concerning their anxiety disorder. This approach, which combines reticence with honesty and disclosure, protects the client's reputation in the community. It is often beneficial to include the prospective spouse in treatment. These issues are illustrated in the following example:

> Mr. E. was a 20-year-old Hasidic man who began treatment after avoiding many opportunities to date. In the initial interview, Mr. E. presented a history of panic disorder with agoraphobia beginning in his late teens. For several years, he had been experiencing anxiety during large gatherings in his synagogue. On several occasions, he had fled the synagogue with panic anxiety. His symptoms led him to return home prematurely from a course of study at an out-of-town *yeshiva*. The impairment caused by his disorder presented a barrier to his personal and professional development.
>
> A focus of treatment was the dating process and strategies for discussing his disorder with a prospective wife. Mr. E. had dated a few women but none had developed into a serious relationship. When he began dating a young woman and they both contemplated marriage, Mr. E. became unsure of how to discuss this with his fiancée. The therapist arranged a joint consultation, with written release from the client, with the prospective spouse. The focus of this consultation, which they both reported was helpful, was to educate them about the course and treatment of anxiety disorders. It was helpful for the therapist to provide information about panic disorder. This included a reassurance that these anxiety symptoms did not prevent the client from being a good husband and father. Indeed, panic disorder did not indicate a grave character defect.
>
> Treatment included a psychoeducational component, teaching of cognitive strategies, relaxation and diaphragmatic breathing training, and *in vivo* exercises. Treatment focused on "real-life issues," which included the commitment to date and strategies to obtain employment. Mr. E. experienced a significant reduction of anxiety during treatment and eventually became engaged and married to the woman who attended the joint session.

HOLIDAYS AND SABBATH

It is recommended that therapists become knowledgeable about the Jewish calendar and the rules, restrictions, and rituals associated with daily events, the Sabbath, and various holidays. The effectiveness of the therapist's work with Orthodox clients will be enhanced by an understanding that these traditional ways, although sometimes time consuming, are a source of joy and provide a sense of continuity for the client and community.

The Sabbath, or day of rest, begins at sundown on Friday and ends an hour after sundown on Saturday. Much of this day of rest is spent in the synagogue with family, praying and studying. It is often the only time during the busy week that the family eats meals together. Meals on the Sabbath and holidays are lengthy and elaborate and include singing, studying, and reviewing religious texts. Worldly activities such as working, driving, using the telephone, or even directly turning on a light are proscribed on the Sabbath. These restrictions can lead to worsening of symptoms for some Orthodox clients with anxiety disorders. For example, an Orthodox Jew is forbidden to carry any object in public on the Sabbath unless it is medically required or unless the community has created an *eruv* (a ritual fence around the neighborhood that creates one large private domain).

Because many Orthodox Jewish communities have not created this *eruv*, members cannot carry objects on the Sabbath. This restriction includes objects that the anxiety-disordered patient might want to carry such as medication, water, or any security object. Despite the risk of heightening social embarrassment or family tension, some agoraphobics may avoid religious services because of this restriction.

Orthodox clients are often concerned that they will be unable to telephone their therapist for reassurance on the Sabbath. When a religious holiday falls immediately before or after the sabbath, a client may not be able to telephone for as many as 3 days. Exceptions can, of course, be made with rabbinical consultation for true medical emergencies. For example, suicidal patients may use the telephone on the Sabbath and seriously medically ill clients may travel by car to a hospital or physician. Anxiety related to these restrictions is shown in the following case example.

Ms. E., an Orthodox woman in her 20s, entered treatment for panic disorder and agoraphobia. Her symptoms began in adolescence with a marked avoidance of school activities such as trips or large social gatherings. Currently, Ms. E. experienced an exacerbation of anxiety, panic attacks, and avoidant behavior in the days before and during the Sabbath and holidays. She feared being cut off from help because she could not travel by car to the hospital or use the telephone. She began to telephone relatives frantically on Friday afternoon seeking reassurance. This pattern of behavior worsened her anxiety as sundown approached and she anticipated an abrupt termination of contact. After the start of Sabbath, she in fact experienced a reduction in anxiety and was able to observe it properly because she accepted that she had no recourse. Although she worried that she would violate Sabbath restrictions by making phone calls, she never actually broke the rules of the Sabbath.

Cognitive-behavioral treatment began with an examination of Ms. E.'s faulty beliefs. She then gradually began attending Sabbath and holiday services, while limiting calls to family for reassurance. Ms. E. agreed to instruct her family that they should not provide this Friday afternoon reassurance. Her anxiety improved as she confronted her fears in therapy and used cognitive strategies and relaxation techniques rather than relying on reassurance from others to manage anxiety. Ms. E. and her therapist prepared a self-help audiotape, made in her own voice. This was used for support during *in vivo* exposure to feared situations.

The lengthy Sabbath and holiday services may promote an urge to flee in many Orthodox Jews with anxiety disorders. Agoraphobics may feel trapped when they are required to remain in the synagogue or visit relatives for a long period of time. Male agoraphobics may avoid participation in important religious practices such as leading prayers or responding to a call to the Torah. Unfortunately, avoidance of a public role generally heightens an Orthodox Jew's sense of poor self-esteem, social isolation and fragility.

Mr. C., previously described, reported that sitting in the synagogue worsened his anxiety and agoraphobic symptoms. Interestingly, his anxiety was greatly reduced when he prayed in a synagogue in which he was *not* a member, because he told himself, "If I leave early, no one knows me or cares." However, the resulting frequent changes in synagogues were stressful for his family. Additionally, his father-in-law assumed that the patient was angry at or insulted by his side of the family because the patient always declined invitations to share holiday meals at their home. Eventually, these avoidance behaviors proved to be an ineffective long-term strategy. After attending a given synagogue for a few weeks, the leaders of the congregation, in a traditional welcoming gesture, asked him to lead services. Refusal of this invitation was socially awkward and anxiety provoking. Cognitive-behavioral treatment, including *in vivo* work to help Mr. C. remain in this phobic situation until his anxiety lessened, was effective, and he was able to return to his synagogue.

RABBINICAL CONSULTATION

In order to enhance the effects of treatment with Orthodox patients, it is often necessary to work collaboratively with a rabbi. A patient might resist a behavioral exercise because of a mistaken belief that it is not religiously permitted. Although a therapist who is educated about Jewish law may be able to recognize and correct any misinterpretations or distortions in Jewish law, it is often necessary to encourage the patient to consult a rabbi of his or her choice. However, particularly when working with patients with obsessive–compulsive disorder, it is important to avoid "rabbi shopping" (Greenberg & Witzum, 1989). Clients are therefore encouraged to agree before the consultation that they will follow the advice of their chosen rabbi. This approach lessens ambiguity and confusion. What follows are some examples of issues in treatment that often need "rabbinical consultation."

Some of the issues involved in obtaining a rabbinical consultation in providing exposure and response prevention treatment with an Orthodox Jew are illustrated in the following case:

> Mr. H., a 40-year-old man, reported a long history of obsessive–compulsive disorder, which began when he was 13 years old. At that time, he recalled being "plagued by doubts whether I had properly recited my prayers." Due to these "doubts," he would compulsively recite for hours prayers that should take a few minutes. Over the years, the nature of his obsessions changed. His rabbi told us he encouraged Mr. H. to present for treatment because "his many concerns regarding preparation for Passover are unrealistic and symptoms of a disorder."
>
> In brief, the patient was always "worried that the food I eat during the year that is *chometz* (leavened bread) may get into some of my belongings and make my house very difficult to clean for Passover." On Passover, Orthodox Jews remove all traces of leavened products from their home. This patient, throughout the year, would be extremely careful where he would sit (i.e., compulsively check to make sure that there was no bread on the chair that could perhaps stick to his pants without his being aware of it).
>
> The nature of the treatment was to encourage him to handle products throughout the year as other members of the community do and to not "respond to his obsessive worries" and engage in extensive rituals such as repetitively washing his hands after every meal to

make sure he "did not spread any crumbs." Initially, the patient was very reluctant to follow the treatment program, but, after consultation with his rabbinical leader, he agreed to a course of intensive exposure and response prevention.

This was aided by having a family session with his wife. She reported that for years she had been trying to get her husband to "not worry so much about these things." She was concerned that his behavior was affecting the children "where he would insist that they wash their hands repetitively after and before meals." Once the treatment alliance was established with the patient, and with the support of his wife, he engaged in exposure and response prevention, and his compulsive rituals dramatically decreased.

The use of a rabbinical consultation is generally encouraged with decisions regarding the use of birth control. Although the therapist should not routinely encourage the Orthodox woman to limit the size of the family, there are cases in which having more children presents a clear and serious risk to the client's mental and physical well-being. In these cases, it is important for the woman to consult with her rabbi. He may counsel that a threat to health temporarily relieves the couple of the obligation of having more children, and therefore the use of contraception is permitted.

Some individuals may misinterpret the rules of fast days such as Yom Kippur or Tishah B'Ab, and may erroneously conclude that everyone in the community is always prohibited from eating or drinking. This is illustrated by a 25-year-old woman who believed that she could not take her prescribed medication on fast days. When her therapist encouraged her to discuss this with her rabbi, the rabbi informed her that she was permitted to take medically essential pills consumed with less than a mouthful of water.

The importance of rabbinical consultation is exemplified in the following case of obsessive–compulsive disorder.

Mr. F., an 18-year-old male with recent onset of abhorrent thoughts (e.g., "I imagine my rabbi as a Nazi"), reported he constantly engaged in mental compulsions to reduce anxiety. He compulsively repeated to himself such self-statements as "I tell myself the rabbi is a *tzadik*" (righteous man). He also avoided prayer and study because he erroneously believed that it was a sin to pray or study Torah while experiencing these thoughts.

Treatment included a variety of components including psychoeducation, as well as exposure and response prevention (Foa, Steketee, & Ozarow, 1985). Mr. F. was encouraged to avoid responding to his obsessions with mental compulsions. He was instructed instead to continue to engage in his normal activities including customary three-times-per-day prayer. He resisted these instructions until he discussed the treatment approach with a respected rabbinical leader. The rabbi explained that obsessions (and his obsessive–compulsive disorder) were not a sin or cause for any change in customary prayers and encouraged Mr. F. to comply with treatment. After the rabbinical consultation, Mr. F. was able virtually to eliminate his compulsions, and eventually his obsessions decreased as well.

Orthodox Jews diagnosed with obsessive–compulsive disorder who experience abhorrent, violent obsessions often experience great concern and guilt about the meaning of these thoughts. For example, they might fear that God will punish them and hold them responsible for their thoughts. On Yom Kippur, the high point of the Ten Days of Repentance, Orthodox Jews believe that they will not be included in the "book of life" (a favorable judgment by God for the coming year) unless they atone for their sins. This holiday may be a time of additional stress for Orthodox Jews with obsessive–compulsive disorder.

> Mr. F., the young man described above, suddenly began doubting on Yom Kippur whether he had completely wiped away all fecal material after a bowel movement. He believed that, because Jewish law prohibits praying unless an individual is "clean," he was required to clean himself thoroughly. He did not participate in prayers or services because he spent much of the day engaged in repetitive washing and checking behaviors. Eventually, he requested advice and a religious ruling from the rabbi who encouraged him to "just wipe once or twice" and return to services immediately thereafter.

Many Orthodox individuals, as part of their religious practice may adapt a *chumrah* (a culturally acceptable, extrastringent religiosity). At times, it is important for the therapist and/or rabbi to work with the client to differentiate between *chumrah* and obsessive–compulsive disorder.

Much of the literature on the treatment of obsessive–compulsive disorder in religious patients has focused on treatment of Orthodox Jews and Roman Catholics (Greenberg & Witztum, 1987; Suess & Halpern, 1987). Orthodox patients often present with certain behaviors such that a therapist unfamiliar with this religious group might have difficulty distinguishing between acceptable religious rituals and obsessive–compulsive disorder symptoms. However, although it may be unclear to the therapist, other Orthodox members of the community such as family members or the rabbi are usually easily able to distinguish between obsessive–compulsive disorder and acceptable religious practices.

The following criteria (Greenberg & Witztum, 1987) are helpful in making this determination:

1. Does the compulsive behavior go far beyond the requirement of religious law?
2. Does the compulsive behavior have a narrow or overly trivial focus? For example, the behavior may focus solely on issues of food purity and not on a full range of religious practices.
3. Are the requirements of work, prayer, and family demands ignored or not receiving enough attention?

It is also important at times to distinguish those patients with obsessive–compulsive disorder from those with psychotic delusions. In general, those suffering with delusions often resist coming to therapy, only agreeing when family members insist. They resist taking the advice of their rabbi and following behavioral treatment or taking medication. These patients must be strongly encouraged to seek pharmacological treatment for their psychotic symptoms.

It is crucial that the therapist not treat patients with exposure to situations proscribed by religious law. For example, patients should never be encouraged to eat nonkosher food. The details of whether an exposure exercise is permitted can be checked with the patient's rabbi.

RELATIONSHIP WITH THE THERAPIST

It is important to be aware of social and political events that may impact upon the Jewish, and particularly the Orthodox Jewish, community. Posttraumatic stress disorder has been extensively studied in recent years among veterans as well as among civilian populations (Jones & Barlow, 1990). Recently, there have been numerous incidents of acts of terrorism affecting Jewish civilian populations around the world. The Crown Heights Lubavitcher community had been exposed to violence in 1991 during which 72 hours of rioting ended with a rabbinical student being knifed to death. At the same time, this community also experienced the stress of the catastrophic stroke and prolonged illness of their charismatic leader, the Rebbe who had led the group for the past 43 years.

On March 1, 1994, a van transporting 15 students ranging in age from 16 to 21 was fired upon on an entrance ramp to the Brooklyn Bridge. This gunman killed one student instantly, and another was critically injured with a bullet wound to the head. A total of approximately 30 shots was fired. In the chaos occurring in the van itself, one student attempted to control the profuse bleeding from the head wound of the student next to him while others lay on the seats or floor of the van. The driver of the van was fired upon numerous times at close range by the gunman using two semiautomatic pistols, who drove in his car alongside the van. In the ensuing chase, two additional students were wounded, with one receiving serious abdominal wounds. Of the original 15 boys in the van, 1 was killed, 1 was critically wounded, and 2 left the country immediately after the shooting.

In a study of the 11 students who were available for evaluation (Trappler & Friedman, 1996), we found that, in contrast to age-matched controls, 4 of the 11 survivors were diagnosed with posttraumatic stress disorder (all comorbid for major depressive disorder), 1 for major depressive disorder, and 2 for adjustment disorder. In spite of intense short-term group work as well as individual work, a 1-year follow-up indicated that the subjects with posttraumatic stress disorder continued to show residual symptomatology. The subjects with depression, anxiety, and adjustment symptoms appeared to be spontaneously resolving and reintegrating socially.

Our clinical experience in working with members of the Orthodox Jewish community of Crown Heights was that many people who were not directly involved in this attack experienced either an increase in their anxiety disorder or experienced clinical symptoms for the first time. It appears that this event "traumatized" many members of the community by leaving them feeling vulnerable and helpless.

It is important for the clinician to be sensitive to the fact that many Orthodox individuals are readily identifiable and vulnerable to antisemitism due to their traditional clothes (men may wear *yarmulkes,* caps to cover their heads). An understanding of these events and their impact upon the individual and community is helpful in establishing rapport with Orthodox patients.

There is individual variability in the choice of therapist. Some ultra-Orthodox individuals may only consult a Orthodox Jewish therapist of the same gender. It is important to discuss these issues in treatment. Other Orthodox individuals may choose to work with either a same or different gender therapist or a non-Jewish therapist, depending on preference or availability. A therapist's experience and reputation in the community is often more important than either religious affiliation or gender.

The therapist's respect for and sensitivity to the cultural and religious values of the Orthodox Jews is essential in building the necessary therapeutic relationship. For example, Orthodox Jews view conservative dress as a sign of respect, and they believe that any physical touching between members of the opposite sex outside marriage is prohibited. The therapist should therefore refrain from touching (including a handshake) a client of the opposite sex. Therapists may likewise choose appropriately conservative dress not for the purpose of "passing" as Orthodox, but to convey respect. Raising the issues and exploring their meaning may be important to the therapeutic relationship. Many Orthodox Jewish clients wonder whether a non-Orthodox therapist understands and respects their values. They are often reluctant to ask the therapist directly and instead may question whether the therapist is Jewish or has experience with working with Orthodox Jews. In our opinion, it is best to answer honestly and directly questions about our ethnic backgrounds and clinical experience. The usual therapeutic stance of inquiring about the meaning of the client's concerns is best left for exploration after directly answering those concerns. Even if we, the therapists, are Jewish, we must not assume that we understand all of the laws and ways of the Orthodox community. Because beliefs and traditions vary among Orthodox Jews, we ask all clients to explain what these laws mean to them and how they believe the laws affect their disorder or treatment.

In general, it is also important to be aware of and sensitive to the effects of anti-Semitism in society. It may be difficult for an Orthodox Jew to trust a therapist from outside of his or her community. It is crucial that therapists examine whether they hold any anti-Semitic beliefs or biases that could affect the outcome of treatment.

CONCLUSIONS

The Orthodox Jewish community has generally been underserved by social service agencies and mental health professionals (Trappler, Greenberg, & Friedman, 1995). Orthodox individuals are generally less interested in long-term or insight-oriented psychotherapy, unless it produces improved functioning in daily living. The primary goal of treatment for most Orthodox clients with anxiety disorders is the elimination or reduction of anxiety symptoms. We have found cognitive-behavioral treatment to be an effective approach for helping Orthodox clients achieve their identified goal (i.e., the development of coping skills that allow them to return to premorbid functioning and to meet the demands of their role in the family and community). This is particularly true for those without severe personality or other Axis I disorders.

Some Orthodox clients are less willing to consider the use of antianxiety and antipanic medications because they often believe that to do so would signify that they have a serious mental illness. However, many individuals respond to encouragement to accept medication and benefit from the combination of medication and cognitive-behavioral treatment. For others, medication is often preferred because they may believe that in a psychotherapeutic treatment their religious values and beliefs may be challenged. Medication may be seen as a more "neutral" treatment.

Mental health professionals need to appreciate the many strengths of individuals from these communities, including strong family support and religious values. It is important to note that the training of many psychotherapists, as well as the development of psychological theories, has often either neglected or been critical of religious beliefs. Writings by Freud, for example, include a description that religion is a "universal obsessional neurosis" (Freud, 1907/1971). It has also been noted that the DSM-IV glossary of technical terms may reveal cultural insensitivity (Larson et al., 1993). Larson and colleagues suggest that the DSM-IV glossary has an excessive focus on religion in illustrating psychopathology. In other words, examples used in psychiatric literature more often focus on the maladaptive qualities of religions rather than on the adaptive functions.

It is essential that the therapist not disrespect or challenge a religious belief unless it is clearly established that the patient has misinterpreted Jewish law. Even then, this challenge is best made after consultation and collaboration with a rabbi. The therapist who has incorporated an understanding for the history and culture and a respect for Jewish laws is able to build a strong working alliance. This knowledge is important in distinguishing between beliefs based on Jewish law, and those based on the faulty cognitions of the patient with an anxiety disorder. The therapist who is educated about the Orthodox Jewish community's values and mores will be better able to offer effective treatment.

SUMMARY

This chapter focused on the cognitive-behavioral treatment of anxiety disorders in Orthodox Jews. Treatment is most effective when therapists are knowledgeable about cultural and religious issues. We provided an overview of the community and reviewed some of the major beliefs and holidays as they affect treatment. Some issues concerning family relations, confidentiality, and consultation with religious leaders were also discussed. Case examples to highlight these issues were presented. The need for culturally sensitive treatment with this group, as well as other religious groups was emphasized. We hope this chapter will stimulate further clinical interest and research.

ACKNOWLEDGMENTS

An earlier version of this chapter was presented at the 14th National Conference of the Anxiety Disorders Association of America, Santa Monica, California, March 1994, as part of a symposium "Diagnosing and Treating Anxiety Disorders: A Multi-Cultural Perspective," Steven Friedman, Ph.D., Chair. This work was supported, in part, by National Institute of Mental Health Grant No. 42545 and by funds from the Department of Psychiatry's Practice Plan at the State University of New York Health Science Center at Brooklyn. The chapter is also adapted from Paradis, Friedman, Hatch, and Ackerman (1996). Copyright 1996 by the Association for Advancement of Behavior Therapy. Adapted by permission of the publisher.

REFERENCES

Academic American Encyclopedia (electronic version). (1993). Danbury, CT: Grolier.

Ackerman, R. (1982). Women's issues in the assessment and treatment of phobias. In R. L. DuPont (Ed.), *Phobia: A comprehensive summary of modern treatments.* New York: Brunner/Mazel.

American Psychiatric Association. (1994). *Diagnostic and statistical manual of mental disorders* (4th ed.). Washington, DC: Author.

Davidson, S. (1980). The clinical effects of massive psychic trauma in families of holocaust survivors. *Journal of Marital and Family Therapy, 6,* 11–20.

Foa, E. B., Steketee, G. S., & Ozarow, B. J. (1985). Behavior therapy with obsessive-compulsives: From theory to treatment. In M. Mavissakalian, S. M. Turner, & L. Michelson (Eds.), *Obsessive–compulsive disorders: Psychological and pharmacological treatment.* New York: Plenum Press.

Freud, S. (1971). Obsessive actions and religious practices. In J. Strachey (Ed. and Trans.), *The standard edition of the complete psychological works of Sigmund Freud* (Vol. 9). London: Hogarth Press. (Original work published 1907)

Friedman, S. (1987). Technical considerations in the behavioral–marital treatment of agoraphobia. *American Journal of Family Therapy, 15,* 112–122.

Friedman, S., Hatch, M. A., Paradis, C. M., Popkin, M., & Shalita, A. R. (1993). Obsessive–compulsive disorder in two black ethnic groups: Incidence in an urban dermatology clinic. *Journal of Anxiety Disorders, 7,* 343–348.

Friedman, S., Paradis, C. M., & Hatch, M. (1994). Characteristics of African American and white patients with panic disorder and agoraphobia. *Hospital and Community Psychiatry, 45,* 798–803.

Gaw, A. C. (1993). *Culture, ethnicity and mental illness.* Washington DC: American Psychiatric Press.

Greenberg, D., & Witztum, E. (1989). The treatment of obsessive–compulsive disorder in strictly religious patients. In J. Rapoport (Ed.), *OCD in children and adolescents.* Washington, DC: American Psychiatric Press.

Hafner, R. J. (1982). The marital context of the agoraphobic syndrome. In D. L. Chambless & A. Goldstein (Eds.), *Agoraphobia: Multiple perspectives on theory and treatment.* New York: Wiley.

Hayes, S. C., & Toarmino, D. (1995). If behavioral principles are generally applicable, why is it necessary to understand cultural diversity? *Behavior Therapist, 18,* 21–23.

Hirsch, S. R. (1967). *The Pentateuch.* New York: Judaica Press.

Horowitz, B. (1993). *The 1991 New York Jewish population study.* United Jewish Appeal—Federation of New York, NY.

Jenkins, J. H. (1994). Culture, emotion and psychopathology. In S. K. Kitayama & H. R. Markus (Eds.), *Emotion and culture: Empirical studies of mutual influence.* Washington, DC: American Psychological Association.

Jones, J. C., & Barlow, D. (1990). The etiology of posttraumatic stress disorder. *Clinical Psychological Review, 10,* 299–328.

Jucovy, M. E. (1992). Psychoanalytic contributions to holocaust studies. *International Journal of Psycho-Analysis, 73,* 267–282.

Larson, D. B., Thielman, S. B., Greenwold, M. A., Lyons, J. S., Post, S. G., Sherrill, K. A., Woods, G. G., & Larson, S. S. (1993). Religious content in the DSM-III glossary of technical terms. *American Journal of Psychiatry, 150,* 1884–1885.

Neighbors, H. W. (1988). The help-seeking behavior of Black Americans. *Journal of the National Medical Association, 80,* 1009–1012.

Ostrov, S. (1978). Sex therapy with Orthodox Jewish couples. *Journal of Sex and Marital Therapy, 4,* 266–278.

Paradis, C. M., Friedman, S., Hatch, M. L., & Ackerman, R. (1996). Cognitive behavioral treatment of anxiety disorders in Orthodox Jews. *Cognitive and Behavioral Practice, 3,* 271–278.

Suess, L., & Halpern, M. S. (1989). Obsessive–compulsive disorder: The religious perspective. In J. Rapoport (Ed.), *OCD in children and adolescents.* Washington, DC: American Psychiatric Press.

Trappler, B., & Friedman, S. (1996). Post-traumatic stress disorder in survivors of the Brooklyn Bridge shooting. *American Journal of Psychiatry, 153,* 705–707.

Trappler, B., Greenberg, S., & Friedman, S. (1995). Treatment of Hassidic Jewish patients in a general hospital medical–psychiatric unit. *Hospital and Community Psychiatry, 46,* 833–835.

Twersky, A. J. (1993). *I am I.* (Available from Mesorah Publications Ltd., Brooklyn, NY, 11223)

8

African Americans

ANGELA M. NEAL-BARNETT
JEFFREY SMITH, SR.

Prior to 1991, few studies existed in the area of anxiety disorders and African Americans. Since that time, a limited amount of new literature has emerged, focusing primarily on panic disorder among adults and fears/phobias in children. In general, the research has been experimental in nature. Limited information is available on anxiety treatment with African Americans, with our review of the literature revealing one treatment study. In this study, a *post hoc* investigation of *in vivo* exposure therapy with agoraphobics, African Americans were found to be more symptomatic and to show less improvement at treatment's end than their white counterparts (Chambless & Williams, 1995).

In this chapter we explore issues in the assessment and treatment of anxiety for African Americans. We begin with a discussion of how this particular ethnic group views mental illness in general and anxiety specifically, and the implications of these views for treatment. Next we investigate the manifestation of the various anxiety disorders in black American populations. The information from these sections forms the basis for our discussion on assessment and treatment issues. We discuss key points in assessing and establishing a working alliance with African American populations, as well as specific needs that must be addressed above and beyond standard treatment when working with anxious African Americans. Because we are clinical researchers and believe strongly in the scientist/practitioner model, we have grounded this paper in the empirical research. Throughout, we give case examples from our own work and the work of our colleagues.

HISTORICAL OVERVIEW

Historically, African Americans have been the targets of misdiagnoses at the hands of the psychological and psychiatric professions (Thomas & Sillen, 1972; Washington, 1994). Records from the antebellum period indicate that Southern white physicians routinely pathologized and misdiagnosed black slave behavior (Guthrie, 1976; Thomas & Sillen, 1972; Williams, 1986). For example, runaway slaves were said to suffer from "drapetomania" or the flight from madness. Based on this diagnosis, rather than fleeing from the oppression of slavery, blacks were fleeing from insanity. Slaves who engaged in oppositional or rebellious behavior were classified as experiencing "dyaesthesis aethiopica" (Thomas & Sillen, 1972). This diagnosis was used to counter charges that slaves' rebellious behavior was due to their dissatisfaction with their condition.

The practice of misdiagnosing African Americans and labeling their logical behavior as deviant extends well into the 20th century. Blacks were frequently misdiagnosed and sent to facilities where their true problem were not discovered for years. The classic case is the North Carolina man who in 1928 was diagnosed as insane and remained institutionalized for over 68 years until it was discovered that he was a deaf–mute ("Deaf Man," 1994). The disability had remained undetected in part because the state of North Carolina taught two versions of sign language, one for whites and one for blacks. Therefore, his sign language was unintelligible to the mental health professionals who made the original diagnosis, and apparently subsequent diagnoses ("Deaf Man," 1994).

Misdiagnoses have not been limited to individual blacks, but have been and continue to be assigned to African American families. Clinicians and academicians have characterized the black family as inferior, disorganized, unstable, and a breeding ground for pathology (Moynihan, 1965; Boyd-Franklin, 1989; Royse & Turner, 1980). Often, the strength of black families and the role of the extended family is ignored.

Misdiagnosis continues today, albeit on a smaller scale than we have seen in the past. African Americans continue to be assigned more severe pathology than their white counterparts who exhibit similar symptoms (Lindsey & Paul, 1989; Neal & Turner, 1991). Capers (1994) and Worthington (1992) suggest that misdiagnosis may be an outcome of racial bias, discrimination, and cultural ignorance. Others have suggested that use of improper assessment tools and failure to use correctly structured interviews may contribute to the problem (Friedman & Paradis, 1991; Neal & Turner, 1991; Neal-Barnett & Smith, 1996). Whether for reasons of cultural ignorance, racial bias, discrimination, insufficient training, lack of structured instruments, or inability of the client/subject to comprehend the question, misdiagnosis still occurs. Currently many clinical researchers acknowledge the tragedy of misdiagnosis and the need for practitioners and researchers to take positive measures in training and assessment to increase accuracy in diagnosis of African Americans (Capers, 1994; Chambless & Williams, 1995; Friedman, Hatch, Paradis, Popkin, & Shalita, 1993; Friedman & Paradis, 1991; Horwath, Johnson, & Horning, 1993; Neal & Turner, 1991; Neal, Nagle-Rich, & Smucker, 1994; Neighbors, 1988; Paradis, Friedman, Lazar, Grubea, & Washington, 1992).

Clearly, with its historical roots and racist overtones, the practice of misdiagnosing African Americans has affected their views of mental illness. But it is not misdiagnosis alone that affects African Americans' conceptualization of mental illness; the documented and perceived mistreatment of African Americans by members of the helping profession also affects views toward mental illness. Once again, a historical examination reveals that low-income blacks often served as subjects for new forms of treatment or no treatment at all. The Tuskegee study, the radium studies, the icepickalon studies, and the Baltimore child care studies represent medical and psychological research where the black participants were misled about the true nature of the treatment (Washington, 1994). Some of these treatments were unsafe and resulted in irreparable damage (Thomas & Sillen, 1972; Washington, 1994). Other treatments, such as behavior therapy, have been seen as brainwashing and ways to control black males (Neal-Barnett & Smith, 1996). Mistreatment by psychologists and psychiatrists has led many African Americans to subscribe to the belief that people who go to a mental health facility are "more crazy after coming out then they were before they went in."

The work experience of one member of our research team in the child welfare system illustrates the legacy of mistrust generated by mistreatment. African American adults whose families are referred or court ordered for treatment often express the belief that their race will prevent them from receiving the best treatment. Assignment to white therapists leads many to surmise that the white therapist cannot relate to their lifestyle, culture, or experience as African Americans. The trepidation and/or anger at being referred or court ordered is heightened by these beliefs, and children often adopt the views of their parents. Whereas most therapists are aware of the anger component, many fail to recognize the mistreatment-fear aspect, thus confirming the client's misgivings about the process. The end result is an unsatisfactory experience for both the client and the therapist.

HELP-SEEKING BEHAVIOR

An analysis of the help-seeking literature sheds further light on African Americans' views of mental illness. Although recent data suggest that African Americans are more likely to use mental health services today than they were 20–25 years ago, the numbers still remain small (Neighbors, Caldwell, Thompson, & Jackson, 1994). Clinical researchers have suggested that those patients seeking relief from physical symptoms tend to use neighborhood health centers and hospital emergency rooms, while those experiencing mental health stressors are more apt to use the informal network established by the family and community. Low-income black females with little or no insurance are more likely to access the informal system than low-income males or middle-class males and females (Block, 1981; Neal & Turner, 1991; Neighbors, 1988; Sue, 1977). Even in instances when support is offset by strain in the family, many African Americans opt not to participate in the mental health system (Chambless & Williams, 1995).

For many African Americans of all economic classes, a significant member of their support system is the black minister. The respect bestowed on clergy members is reflected in the titles they are assigned by their congregations—pastor, shepherd, elder. Implicit in these titles are acts of fearless protection and advocacy, unconditional acceptance, a spirit of untiring forgiveness, and the ability to teach and instruct toward correction. Many parishioners see their pastors as people "called by God" and therefore attribute God-like qualities to those individuals. The messages conveyed in spiritual songs and sermons may serve to foster dependence on a minister rather than on a mental health professional. Songs such as *God Will Take Care of You* (W. S. Martin & Martin, 1977), *Precious Lord, Take My Hand* (Dorsey, 1939/1977), *I Must Tell Jesus* (Hoffman, 1977), *Peace in the Valley* (Dorsey, 1939/1977), *What a Friend We Have in Jesus* (Converse & Scriven, 1977), *Sweet Hour of Prayer* (Bradbury & Walford, 1977), and *Just a Little Talk with Jesus* (Derricks, 1937/1977) encourage reliance on the Lord and his emissaries. Research and our experience indicate that some African American clergy actively discourage their members from seeking help from "Godless" professionals, whereas others encourage their parishioners to use the services of psychologists, psychiatrists, and counselors

(Lyles, 1992). On multiple occasions, we have heard ministers ridicule psychologists. Our favorite is the minister who repeatedly told his parishioners, "I studied psychology in college, I know what psychologists do." In contrast, we are invited frequently to speak at black churches on anxiety and fear. These invitations have led to us providing consultation to several ministers in establishing referral lists, counseling programs, and health ministries.

Scant literature exists that focuses exclusively on the help-seeking behavior of the black middle class. Are their views of mental illness and the help-seeking behavior similar to those of their working- and lower-class counterparts? To answer this question, we must first understand who the black middle class are. Middle-class African Americans are divided into two distinct groups, multigenerational and first-generation middle class (Cose, 1993; Edwards & Polite, 1992). Prior to the Civil Rights movement, many jobs were closed to African Americans. Therefore individuals in the multigenerational group are just as likely to be the children or grandchildren of Pullman porters, teachers, farmers, and undertakers as they are to be the children of doctors and lawyers. For African Americans, middle-class attainment is predicated more on education than economics. The reason for the heightened emphasis on education is that African Americans with comparable degrees routinely earn less than their white counterparts. Whereas middle class status for white couples appears predicated on one income, for black couples two incomes are often necessary. Only 7.5% of African American's households income equals or exceeds $50,000 (Boston, 1996). Many middle-class African Americans are employed in predominantly white settings, and experience institutional racism on a regular basis. Later in this chapter we will discuss the possible role of institutional racism in the development of anxiety disorders.

The available information indicates that middle-class African Americans do not routinely seek help from mental health professionals. Rather, middle-class African Americans, particularly African American women, are actively participating in self-help groups. These groups, more commonly known as "sister circles," take place in homes, churches, bookstores, and schools. The central themes of sister circles appear to be affirmation, self-recovery, and healing. Guidebooks in this process include *In the Company of My Sisters* (Boyd, 1993), *Value in the Valley* (Vanzant, 1993), *In the Spirit* (Taylor, 1993), and *Sisters of the Yam* (hooks, 1993). As indicated by the guidebooks' titles, spirituality is an important aspect of the groups.

Middle-class black males appear less likely than middle-class black females to seek help or engage in self-help. In addition to the historical reasons, black males perceive therapy as something to be shunned or ashamed of (Johnson, 1995). To procure black males' participation in couples therapy, some psychologists frame it as a way of helping the spouse or significant other (Johnson, 1995). By using this approach, the therapist is appealing to the black male's inherent sense of power and *machismo* (Johnson, 1995).

African Americans' views of mental illness and therapy, as well as their help-seeking behavior, appear to affect their conceptualization of fear and anxiety. The views of many African American males about anxiety are neatly illustrated in the words of Langston Hughes's character Jess B. Semple:

> In my time I have been cut, stabbed, run over, hit by a car, tromped by a horse, robbed, fooled, deceived, double-crossed, dealt seconds, and mighty near blackmailed—but I am still here! I have been laid off, fired and not rehired, Jim Crowed, segregated, insulted, eliminated, locked in, locked out, locked up, left holding the bag, and denied relief. I have been caught in the rain, caught in jails, caught short with my rent and caught with the wrong woman—but I am still here! My mama should have named me Job instead of Jess B. Semple. I have been underfed, underpaid, undernourished, and everything but undertaken—yet I am still here. The only thing I am afraid of now—is that I will die before my time. (Hughes, 1968, p. 106)

Although Semple's statements may seem exaggerated, many middle-class, working-class, and low-income African American males identify with his statement. Given all the black male must endure, anxiety is the least of his concerns. However, one should not interpret this statement to mean that African American males do not get anxious. What appears to occur is that they do not connect the emotions and cognitions with anxiety and may instead associate them with anger or as being part of life.

Our National Institute of Mental Health-funded work with anxious middle-class African American women indicates that many do not acknowledge their anxiety related emotions. Further investigation suggests that this is a conscious choice. We hypothesize that, for these women, acknowledging anxiety-related emotions is counterproductive. Thus, in a sense, these women are engaging in adaptive behavior. To acknowledge anxiety-related feelings is to admit to feelings and cognitions that may impede one's ability to function, and also may lead to admission of other negatively associated feelings as well (Neal-Barnett, Peoples-Dukes, & Robbins-Brinson, 1996).

Our work with African American women also suggests that there exists a group of women who recognize their anxiety but continue to function and do not seek help. Their failure to seek help does not appear to be related to the factors listed earlier. These women seem to have internalized the stereotype of the strong black women who bears all (Bell-Scott, 1982). Whereas these women continue to function, they readily admit their functioning is somewhat impaired, indicating treatment could be beneficial. Yet they decline therapy, opting instead to rely on either faith, friends, family, intoxicating substances, or some combination thereof.

Many African Americans do not appear to be aware of how anxiety disorders are manifested. Anxiety may not be as recognizable as other disorders such as depression, schizophrenia, or conduct disorder which have very clear-cut symptoms that are visible to family members and outsiders. Neal and Turner (1991) have suggested that certain aspects of African American life may cause symptoms to go undetected. For example, they cite the case of the African American agoraphobic for whom the presence of an extended family network provides the agoraphobic with a number of "safe" individuals allowing the avoidance behavior to go unnoticed (Neal & Turner, 1991, p. 408).

In our practice we do a great deal of anxiety education and prevention work in African American communities and institutions. At a program's conclusion we are frequently approached by individuals who tell us, "I think I might have that" or "Thank you, now I know I'm not crazy" (Neal-Barnett et al., 1996). These responses appear to indicate lack of awareness about anxiety and also association of anxiety symptoms with more severe psychopathology. Research with African American children further illustrates this point. Neal and Ward-Brown (1994) report that low-income, rural African American parents may misinterpret their child's anxious behavior as bad or oppositional behavior.

African Americans also may misinterpret anxiety symptoms as indicative of a physical disorder. Neal et al. (1995) found that individuals with full-blown panic attacks believed the phenomena to be part of their hypertension and therefore did not report the symptoms to their physicians. Friedman and colleagues (1993) found that African American obsessive–compulsive disorder patients were routinely being seen in a dermatology clinic, indicating that the resulting skin condition may have been perceived as more problematic than the compulsive behavior.

In the preceding section we have discussed how anxiety is viewed in various African American communities. We now discuss the specific diagnoses and information available on anxiety disorders in African

American populations. For the purpose of this chapter, we limit our discussion to panic disorder with or without agoraphobia, obsessive–compulsive disorder, social anxiety, and generalized anxiety disorder.

PANIC DISORDER

Panic disorder is defined in the fourth edition of the *Diagnostic and Statistical Manual of Mental Disorders* (DSM-IV) as the presence of recurrent, unexpected panic attacks, followed by at least 1 month of persistent concern over having another panic attack. During one of the attacks, the individual must experience at least four of the following symptoms: palpitations, sweating, trembling or shaking, shortness of breath, feeling of choking, chest pain, nausea, dizziness, depersonalization, fear of losing control, fear of dying, numbness and tingling sensations, or hot flushes or chills. Panic disorder without agoraphobia is diagnosed twice as often as panic disorder with agoraphobia, and women experience it three times more than men (American Psychiatric Association, 1994).

As mentioned earlier in this chapter, among African Americans panic disorder appears to co-occur frequently with hypertension (Neal et al., 1994; Neal & Turner, 1991). This observation, coupled with the fact that hypertension has reached epidemic proportions in the African American community, suggests that black hypertensives may need to be screened for the presence of panic. Our work in medical clinics suggests that some African American hypertensives are misattributing their panic symptoms as hypertension symptoms. As a result, the panic goes untreated and the hypertension remains unchanged.

Research has also uncovered the presence of isolated sleep paralysis among African Americans with panic disorder and hypertension (Bell, Hildreth, Jenkins, & Carter, 1988). Isolated sleep paralysis is a condition that occurs just upon awakening or when falling asleep. During this period, the individual is unable to move the body and may experience vivid hallucinations or feelings of acute danger. When the paralysis subsides, the individual experiences panic-like symptoms. African Americans commonly refer to the disorder as the "the witch is riding you" (Bell, Hildreth, et al., 1988). Among other racial and ethnic groups within and outside the United States, isolated sleep paralysis generally occurs once in a lifetime. However, among African Americans the disorder is recurrent. Because isolated sleep paralysis co-occurs with panic, some researchers have suggested that it might be a different manifestation of the disorder. Another possibility is that isolated sleep paralysis is distinct but serves as a precursor to panic (Neal et al., 1994).

Our experience indicates clients are loathe to talk about their isolated sleep paralysis experiences. This may be due in part to the fact that the experience is profoundly disturbing and that to some it has supernatural overtones. When we inquire about the experience, individuals' voice tone and facial expressions visibly change. Many express that we are the first people they have told about the experience.

As a result of the tendency to misattribute panic symptoms, the hesitancy to talk about isolated sleep paralysis, and the general pattern of help-seeking behavior, many African Americans with panic disorder go untreated for years By the time treatment is sought, many have developed ingrained patterns of avoidance that meet diagnostic criteria for agoraphobia. In addition, comorbid anxiety disorders may also exist, which are generally manifested as specific phobias (Neal-Barnett et al., 1996). The comorbidity rate with nonanxiety disorders such as alcohol abuse, schizophrenia, and major depression is also high (Horwath et al., 1993).

Research indicates that African American panic patients, although they show some improvement, respond less favorably to cognitive-behavioral treatment than whites (Friedman & Paradis, 1991; Chambless & Williams, 1995). The duration of the disorder, the comorbidity with other emotional disorders, and the association with a medical disorder may be contributing factors to the treatment response. Failure to incorporate aspects of African American culture may also play a role. The extended family and fictive kin, failure to consider the context in which the person is living, and failure to incorporate the person's spirituality may make a difference in the treatment response (Neal-Barnett & Smith, 1996). We will expand on these issues in the assessment section of this chapter.

GENERALIZED ANXIETY DISORDER

Generalized anxiety disorder is defined as excessive worry occurring more days than not for a period of at least 6 months where the individual finds it difficult to control the worry. Three of the following six symptoms must accompany the worry: restlessness, easily fatigued, difficulty concentrating, irritability, muscle tension, and/or disturbed sleep. The worry and associated symptoms usually impair social, occupational, and interpersonal functioning. The disturbance cannot be directly caused by drug abuse, medication, or other physiological and medical conditions. Often persons experiencing generalized anxiety disorder complain of muscle tension and soreness; trembling; an unsettled feeling; dry mouth; cold, clammy hands; nausea; urinary frequency; an exaggerated startle response; and depressive-type symptoms (American Psychiatric Association, 1994). Although in clinical settings women present for generalized anxiety disorder more than men, it is believed that the disorder is proportionately equal among the two genders.

Little is known about generalized anxiety disorder among African Americans. As with most anxiety disorders discussed in this chapter, African Americans are conspicuously absent from the literature. The physical tension aspect of the disorder suggests blacks with generalized anxiety disorder may be seen in primary care facilities. Our research teams' work in these facilities suggests that physicians identify patients as anxious, but do not elaborate as to the specific anxiety disorder. Recently, we investigated the presence of anxiety disorders among patients at an internal medicine clinic. Given the physicians' notes, we speculated that the patients characterized as anxious patients might be experiencing the pervasive anxiety associated with generalized anxiety disorder. However, our structured interviews with the patients did not support our hypothesis. Patients were more likely to endorse panic or posttraumatic stress disorder symptoms than generalized anxiety disorder. We must caution that the internal medicine clinic was a training center serving low-income and indigent clients, which may have affected our findings.

Given perceptions of anxiety in African American communities, our experience in the medical setting, and the dearth of literature, the question arises as to whether African Americans experience generalized anxiety disorder. African American folkwit tells us that "worry is a luxury black folks can't afford." Some African Americans may simply experience life in this culture as generalized anxiety disorder, learning to cope with it and continue through life, whereas others, particularly the upwardly mobile, may experience and meet criteria for generalized anxiety disorder as they attempt to balance having "a foot in both worlds" (Dubois, 1902/1970; McLain, 1986). Yet, our interviews with middle-income African American women do not confirm this latter supposition. In particular, we have talked with several women who appear to exhibit generalized anxiety disorder tendencies, but upon careful assessment do not meet diagnostic criteria. Within our research and experience, African Americans rarely endorse generalized anxiety disorder symptomatology.

SOCIAL ANXIETY

Social anxiety among African Americans has seldom been studied. Research with black children has noted the absence of a socioevaluative factor on the Fear Survey Schedule for Children—Revised (Neal, Lilly, & Zakis, 1993). This finding suggests that socioevaluative fears for African American children may not be tapped by standard instruments.

Our own research and clinical experience show that African American children and adults are more likely to experience social anxiety in the presence of other blacks than in the presence of whites. We conducted interviews with socially anxious African American women that revealed that the anxiety is more likely to occur in the presence of other African Americans. These interviews reveal that, at some point in their lives, the women have been accused of "acting white," suggesting that their failure to meet some mythical black standard and, therefore, not fitting in may be the origin of the social anxiety.

Further support for the contention that African Americans are more likely to experience social anxiety in the presence of same-race individuals can be found in our work with children (Neal & Ward-Brown, 1994). Black children were found to experience significantly higher increases in blood pressure when reading aloud to a black audience than when reading aloud to a white audience (Neal & Ward-Brown, 1994).

This perceived tendency for African Americans to be less likely to experience social anxiety in the presence of whites may have historical and developmental roots. America has a long history of racism and many African Americans have developed adaptive ways of coping with this phenomena. The development process of racial socialization (Peters, 1985) has also instilled in many African Americans the ability to deal effectively with whites. When African Americans enter predominantly white situations, the idea that "everyone is watching me" may not be irrational. However, rather than exhibit anxiety, African Americans may activate their learned survival skills, which may manifest themselves in the form of cautious, reserved behavior ("Are Blacks More or Less Shy," 1996) and be misinterpreted as social anxiety.

Some African Americans do experience social anxiety in the presence of whites. Our experience and research suggest that, for some, this type of social anxiety may be a direct offshoot of racism. A common adage instilled in many African Americans at an early age is that one must be "twice as good to go half as far." Whereas belief in this adage may sustain and motivate some, for others it may produce anger, and for still others undue pressure, fear, and anxiety. Many African American professionals have had the institutional racist experience of being perceived as the affirmative action recipient (Carter, 1991). Implicit in this perception is a socioevaluative judgment. We find that some African Americans internalize this message and begin to exhibit behavior and symptoms associated with social anxiety. We have worked with several students and professionals whose performance and/or grades have suffered due to this type of socioevaluative anxiety. For these individuals the core fear appears to be fear of failure and this fear includes failing the extended family and failing the black race. Given the extensive nature of the fear, it is important to build racial coping skills and racial coping statements into the cognitive-behavioral therapy. Failure to tap into the crucial element of racism may hinder treatment progress.

OBSESSIVE–COMPULSIVE DISORDER

According to DSM-IV (American Psychiatric Association, 1994), obsessive–compulsive disorder is defined as persistent, recurrent ideas, thoughts, impulses, or images that are experienced as intrusive, inappropriate, and cause marked anxiety or distress. The disorder is also highlighted by repetitive behaviors (e.g., hand washing, ordering, checking, praying, counting, or repeating words silently) or mental acts in which the goal is to prevent or reduce anxiety or distress, and not to provide pleasure or gratification. The individual may realize that the thoughts and actions are excessive and/or unreasonable, yet may be incapable of resisting. The obsession and compulsion must cause marked distress, be time consuming (take more than one hour per day), or significantly interfere with or disrupt the individual's daily routine, occupational functioning, social activities, relationships with others, or some combination thereof. This disorder is equally found in men and women (American Psychiatric Association, 1994). As previously mentioned, African Americans with obsessive–compulsive disorder are primarily seen in dermatology clinics, indicating it is the secondary medical condition rather than the disorder itself for which African Americans seek help (Friedman et al., 1993). African Americans seeking help from the dermatology clinic were found to be symptomatically similar to white obsessive–compulsive disorder patients presenting at an anxiety disorder clinic (Friedman et al., 1993).

Given our discussion on the anxiety disorders, it should be clear that standard assessment interviews and structured interview schedules may not provide the information necessary to assess anxiety in

African American populations. In our research, we have modified and empirically validated a structured interview for use with African American populations. We have done so because the traditional research does not allow us to examine aspects of African American culture that may be important for assessment and treatment of anxiety disorders. Specifically, as part of our routine assessment we gather information about the extended family, spirituality, isolated sleep paralysis, victimization, and exposure to violence (Neal, 1992). Besides including the aforementioned sections, we have amended the anxiety disorders questions. For example, based on our research, we have amended the panic disorder section to emphasize "the phenomena occur for no reason at all." Based on socioevaluative anxiety data, we routinely inquire if it is easier to perform before people of the same or different race (Neal, 1992).

ISSUES IN ASSESSMENT

Spirituality

Spirituality is a core aspect of African American culture (Hale-Benson, 1986; Rodgers, 1994). Many African Americans, whether or not they participate in an organized religion, have strong convictions about spiritual power and believe in something or someone greater than themselves. Spirituality questions assist our research team in making appropriate diagnoses. Information about an individual's spirituality is crucial in ruling out psychosis. Questions about prophecy, gifts, root work, and hoodoo (the African American version of voodoo) enable the interviewer to clarify information about hallucinations and visions.

We recall a situation where a parent indicated to her therapist that she (parent) was filled with the Holy Spirit and could rid her acting-out daughter of her devilish ways by the laying on of hands. Upon hearing these statements, the therapist diagnosed the mother as delusional and a risk to the teen's safety. Furthermore, she recommended that the child be removed immediately from the mother's home. Fortunately, a professional familiar with the spiritual concept of laying on of hands intervened. The spiritual belief was explained, the situation reassessed, and the recommendation rescinded. However, the parent's and teen's mistrust of the therapist was intensified and the family discontinued services. The inclusion of spirituality as part of the initial assessment would have revealed the mother's grounding in the Pentecostal faith.

Armed with this knowledge, the therapist might have recognized that the mother's laying on of hands was in accordance with the Biblical Scriptures and not a symptom of her mental status.

Spirituality questions also assist us in designing cognitive interventions. In our work with anxious patients, we find Scriptures can be used to counter fallacious cognitions. For the phobia or panic patient, the cognition "I can't do this, I'm too scared" could be replaced with the simple Bible verse "I can do all things through Christ who strengthens me" (Philippians 14:3).

Extended Family

The extended family is an integral part of black American's lives (E. P. Martin & Martin, 1978). The extended family is defined as a multigenerational, independent kinship system that is held together by a sense of obligation to relatives, is organized around a "family-base household," is generally guided by a "dominant family figure," extends across geographical boundaries to connect family units to an extended family network, and has a built-in mutual aid system for the welfare of its members and the maintenance of the family as a whole (E. P. Martin & Martin, 1978, p. 1). These extended kinship networks and the additional social support derived from such networks may serve to insulate the African American anxiety patient. Alternatively, the existence of such networks may inhibit help-seeking behavior because of the extensive support.

Kinship network questions provide information about the household, socioeconomic status, parenting status, and social support. Based on standard sociodemographic questionnaires, an unmarried woman with children may be classified as a single parent. Kinship questions, including "Who lives in your household?", may reveal the presence of grandparents, aunts, uncles, or a long-time companion. Understanding who a person's family is has implications for interventions. Research has found that the identification and involvement of extended family members is integral to the successful treatment of African American panic patients (Friedman & Paradis, 1991).

Victimization and Covictimization

One variable worthy of attention in the assessment of anxiety disorders among blacks is previous exposure to violence and subsequent development of anxiety symptoms. From the basic learning literature we know that prior exposure to fearful stimuli can "prime" one to react fearfully to other stimuli. Thus, the effects of repeated traumatic conditioning experiences can be cumulative (Mineka, 1985). Violence and victimization may be considered traumatic events.

The witnessing of violent acts and victimization are particularly harsh realities in some black communities. African American men, women, and children are more likely to be the victims of a crime than are their white counterparts. They also are more likely than white Americans to know someone who has been the victim of a crime (Bell, 1987; Bell, Taylor-Crawford, Jenkins, & Chalmers, 1988). Victimization screenings at inner-city mental health and primary health care centers have revealed that a significant percentage of those seeking services had been victimized (Bell, Taylor-Crawford, et al., 1988). Neal and Ward-Brown (1994), in a study of anxious black children and their parents, found that these children experienced significantly more traumatic events than their nonanxious black counterparts.

Victimization is not limited to inner-city residents. African Americans, regardless of socioeconomic status, are twice as likely as their white counterparts to witness violence (Neal & Turner, 1991). In our work with middle-class African American women we routinely hear victimization stories. These stories, remarkably similar in content, appear to be directly related to the anxiety disorder exhibited.

THE THERAPEUTIC ALLIANCE

During workshops and presentations, we are frequently asked if non-African American therapists can treat anxious African American clients? Our answer to this question is yes. However, it is crucial that the therapists have a working knowledge and understanding of African American culture. In addition, therapists must understand issues pertinent to low-income, working-class, and middle-class African Americans, yet, at the same time understand that African Americans are not monolithic—that is, there is a great deal of intragroup variety. Becoming culturally sensitive to the needs and issues of African American clients requires time and commitment on the part of the therapist. We are reminded of the comedian Martin Lawrence's routine on whites and cultural sensitivity. In explaining why he refuses to go to predominantly white parties, he says, "Every time I go, some white person gets me in a corner and says, 'Martin, I saw 'Boyz N the Hood.' 'I understand, man, I understand' " (Lawrence, 1993). Lawrence's comments emphasize the idea that viewing a film, reading a book, or reading this chapter is only the beginning. Developing the skills to work with African American clients is a process. Increasing one's knowledge and understanding of African Americans reduces the likelihood that one will approach working with this clientele not from a deficit model but instead by accentuating clients' strengths and assets.

Interaction and experience with African American clients facilitates one's knowledge base and enhances one's skills (Neal-Barnett & Smith, 1996). Many non-African American therapists express concern over how they may be viewed or whether they will be accepted by African American clients. These concerns can impede the therapeutic relationship. Interaction assists the therapist in confronting the concerns. Gaining experience with African American clients may require the practicing clinician to step outside his or her clinic, practice, or university-based center and establish collaborations or consultation with institutions and therapists that serve predominantly black clients or are located in Black communities. Neal and Turner (1991) offer insight as to how these collaborations might be accomplished; the reader is encouraged to follow their suggestions.

For a variety of reasons, many black clients request African American therapists. Some clients may perceive non-African Americans as being insensitive and ignorant of black issues and culture. Others, for historical and personal reasons, have a healthy mistrust of non-African American therapists. An individual's stage in the racial identity process may be a motivating factor. Individuals in the immersion/emersion stage are more likely to request a black therapist (Helms, 1985; Parham, 1989). Upon being assigned to a non-African American therapist, some clients may express disappointment, outrage, or disgust and may passively or actively refuse to participate. In these cases it is important for the therapist and the client to work through the client's perception of the therapist in the initial stages of therapy (Parham, 1989). Failure to do so may impede progress or result in premature termination.

Respect is an important aspect of the therapeutic alliance. Clients who believe their therapist does not respect them are more likely to discontinue treatment. Respect is a key motivating factor for African Americans, particularly males, and little tolerance is expressed for individuals who "diss" (slang for disrespect) them. Some therapists unwittingly display disrespect to their African American clients by calling them by their first name or by calling them out of their name (using the wrong name) (Neal, 1985). When working with adult African American clients, it is important to address them initially as Ms., Mrs., Miss, or Mr. and surname. This caveat is particularly important for therapists working with older African Americans or families. Respect for elders is a hallmark of African American culture. To call an older person by their first name or nickname is considered disgraceful. When working with families, to call adults by their first names is perceived as placing them at the same level as the child(ren) and conveys little respect for their roles as parents. Equally as important as using surnames is to pronounce an individual's name correctly. Many black names are distinctive, are spelled phonetically, and have African roots. For these reasons, they are often mispronounced by people unfamiliar with the culture. A simple solution is to ask the client how to pronounce the name or if one is pronouncing the name correctly. The name issue may sound unimportant, but on more than one occasion we have seen individuals who complained that their previous therapist called them by their first name or "didn't even know their name."

CONCLUSION

In this chapter we have discussed issues germane to the understanding and treatment of anxiety disorders in African American populations. We have presented relevant information based on the available research and our clinical experience. Clearly, the need exists for more published clinical research on anxious African Americans. The effective treatment of anxiety disorders in African Americans begins with the therapist's willingness to develop a working knowledge of the joys and concerns of being black in America. Information concerning racism, perceptions of mental illness, help-seeking behavior, and African American families contributes to the therapist's knowledge and understanding of effective treatment for anxious African Americans.

ACKNOWLEDGMENTS

Work on this chapter was supported in part by Grant No. MH 49557 from the National Institute of Mental Health awarded to Angela M. Neal. The authors would like to thank Nina Goosby for her assistance with this chapter.

REFERENCES

American Psychiatric Association. (1994). *Diagnostic and statistical manual of mental disorders* (4th ed.). Washington, DC: Author.

Are Blacks more or less shy than other races? (1996, April 8). *Jet*, pp. 14–17.

Bell, C. C. (1987). Preventive strategies for dealing with violence among Blacks. *Community Mental Health Journal, 23*, 217–228.

Bell, C. C., Hildreth, C. J., Jenkins, E. J., & Carter, C. (1988). The relationship of isolated sleep paralysis and panic disorder to hypertension. *Journal of the National Medical Association, 80,* 289–294.

Bell, C. C., Taylor-Crawford, K., Jenkins, E. J., & Chalmers, D. (1988). Need for victimization screening in a Black psychiatric population. *Journal of the National Medical Association, 80,* 41–48.

Bell-Scott, P. (1982). Debunking Sapphire. In G. Hull, P. Bell-Scott, & B. Smith (Eds.), *But some of us are brave* (pp. 85–92). Old Westbury, NY: Feminist Press.

Block, C. B. (1981). Black Americans and the cross-cultural counseling and psychotherapy experience. In A. J. Marsella & P. B. Pederson (Eds.), *Cross-culture and psychotherapy* (pp. 177–194). New York: Pergamon Press.

Boston, K. (1996). Building wealth. *Emerge, 7*(6), 51–55.

Boyd, J. A. (1993). *In the company of my sisters.* New York: Dutton.

Boyd-Franklin, N. (1989). *Black families in therapy: A multisystems approach.* New York: Guilford Press.

Branbury, W. B., & Walford, W. W. (1977). Sweet hour of prayer. In *The New National Baptist Hymnal.* Nashville: National Baptist Publishing Board.

Capers, C. F. (1994). Mental health issues and African-Americans. *Nursing Clinics of North America, 29*(1), 57–64.

Carter, S. L. (1991). *Reflections of an affirmative action baby.* New York: Basic Books.

Chambless, D. L., & Williams, K. E. (1995). A preliminary study of African Americans with agoraphobia: Symptom severity and outcome of treatment with in vivo exposure. *Behavior Therapy, 26,* 501–515.

Converse, C. C., & Scriven, J. (1977). What a friend we have in Jesus. In *The New National Baptist Hymnal.* Nashville: National Baptist Publishing Board.

Cose, E. (1993). *The rage of a privileged class.* New York: HarperCollins.

Deaf man, 96, believed to be mentally ill; released from hospital wards after 68 years. (1994, February 21). *Jet,* p. 52.

Derricks, C. (1977). Just a little talk with Jesus. In *The New National Baptist Hymnal* (p. 298). Nashville: National Baptist Publishing Board. (Original work published 1937)

Dorsey, T. A. (1977). Peace in the valley. In *The New National Baptist Hymnal* (p. 44b). Nashville: National Baptist Publishing Board. (Original work published 1939)

Dorsey, T. A. (1977). Precious Lord, take my hand. In *The New National Baptist Hymnal* (p. 339). Nashville: National Baptist Publishing Board. (Original work published 1939)

Dubois, W. E. B. (1902/1970). *The souls of Black folks.* New York: Washington Square Press.

Edwards, A., & Polite, C. (1992). *Children of the dream: The psychology of Black success.* New York: Doubleday.

Friedman, S., Hatch, M., Paradis, C. M., Popkin, M., & Shalita, A. R. (1993). Obsessive–compulsive disorder in two Black ethnic groups: Incidence in an urban dermatology clinic. *Journal of Anxiety Disorders, 7*, 343–348.

Friedman, S., & Paradis, C. (1991). African-American patients with panic disorder and agoraphobia. *Journal of Anxiety Disorders, 5*, 35–41.

Gutherie, R. (1976). *Even the rat was white.* New York: Harper & Row.

Hale-Benson, J. (1986). *Black children: Their roots, culture and learning styles* (rev. ed.). Baltimore: Johns Hopkins Press.

Helms, J. E. (1985). Toward theoretical explanations of the effects of race on counseling: A Black and White model. *Counseling Psychologist, 12*(4), 153–165.

Hoffman, E. A. (1977). I must tell Jesus. In *The New National Baptist Hymnal* (p. 232). Nashville: National Baptist Publishing Board. (Original work published 1939)

hooks, b. (1993). *Sisters of the yam.* Boston: South End Press.

Horwath, E., Johnson, J., & Hornig, C. D. (1993). Epidemiology of panic disorder in African Americans. *American Journal of Psychiatry, 150*(3), 465–469.

Hughes, L. (1968). Census. In A. Chapman (Ed.), *Black voices* (pp. 105–106). New York: New American Library.

Johnson, R. S. (1995). Keeping secrets. *Essence, 26*(7), 19–92.

Lawrence, M. (Executive Producer). (1993, November). *Martin.* Los Angeles: Yougoboy Productions.

Lindsey, K. P., & Paul, G. L. (1989). Involuntary commitments to public mental institutions: Issues involving the over-representation of Blacks and assessment of relevant functioning. *Psychological Bulletin, 106*(2), 171–183.

Lyles, M. (1992). Mental health perceptions of Black pastors: Implications for psychotherapy with Black patients. *Journal of Psychology and Christianity 11*(4), 366–377.

Martin, E. P., & Martin, J. M. (1978). *The Black extended family.* Chicago: University of Chicago Press.

Martin, W. S., & Martin, C. D. (1977). God will take care of you. In *The New National Baptist Hymnal* (p. 220). Nashville: National Baptist Publishing Board. (Original work published 1905)

McGoldrick, M., Pearce, J. K., & Giordano, J. (Eds.). (1982). *Ethnicity and family therapy.* New York: Guilford Press.

McLain, L. (1986). *A foot in each world: Essays and articles by Leanita McLain.* Evanston, IL: Northwestern University Press.

Mineka, S. (1985). The frightful complexity of the origins of fears. In F. R. Bruch & J. R. Overmeier (Eds.), *Affect, conditioning, and cognition: Essays on the determinants of behavior* (pp. 55–73). Hillsdale, NJ: Erlbaum.

Moniyhan, D. P. (1965). *The Negro family: The case for national action.* Washington, DC: U.S. Department of Labor.

Neal, A. M. (1985). *The impact of African American names on perceptions of competence.* Unpublished master's thesis, DePaul University, Chicago, IL.

Neal, A. M. (1992). *ADIS-R adapted for use with Black populations: Revision for use with African American populations.* Kent, OH: Kent State University.

Neal, A. M., Lilly, R. S., & Zakis, S. (1993). What are African American children afraid of? *Journal of Anxiety Disorders, 7,* 129–139.

Neal, A. M., Nagle-Rich, L., & Smucker, W. D. (1994). The presence of panic disorder among African American hypertensives: A pilot study. *Journal of Black Psychology, 20*(1), 29–35.

Neal, A. M., & Turner, S. M. (1991). Anxiety disorders research with African Americans: Current status. *Psychological Bulletin, 109*(3), 400–410.

Neal, A. M., & Ward-Brown, B. J. (1994). Fears and anxiety disorders in African American children. In S. Friedman (Ed.). *Anxiety disorders in African Americans* (pp. 65–75). New York: Springer.

Neal-Barnett, A. M., Peoples-Dukes, J. L., & Robbins-Brinson, L. (1996, May). *Anxiety disorder and hypertension: What you don't know might hurt you.* Workshop presented at Marrow of Tradition, Akron, OH.

Neal-Barnett, A. M., & Smith, J. (1996). African American children and behavioral therapy: Considering the Afrocentric approach. *Cognitive and Behavioral Practice, 3,* 351–369.

Neighbors, H. W. (1985a). Professional help use among Black Americans: Implications for unmet need. *American Journal of Community Psychology, 12,* 551–566.

Neighbors, H. W. (1985b). Seeking professional help for personal problems: Black Americans' use of health and mental health services. *Community Mental Health Journal, 21,* 156–166.

Neighbors, H. W. (1988). The help-seeking behavior of Black Americans. *Journal of the National Medical Association, 80*(9), 1009–1012.

Neighbors, H. W., Caldwell, C. H., Thompson, E., & Jackson, J. S. (1994). Help-seeking behavior and unmet need. In S. Friedman (Ed.), *Anxiety disorders in African Americans* (pp. 26–39). New York: Springer.

Paradis, C. M., Friedman, S., Lazar, R. M., Grubea, J., & Kesselman, M. (1992). Use of a structured interview to diagnose anxiety disorders in a minority population. *Hospital and Community Psychiatry, 43*(1), 61–64.

Parham, T. (1989). Cycles of psychological nigrescence. *Counseling Psychologist, 17*(2), 187–226.

Peters, M. F. (1985). Racial socialization of young Black children. In H. P. McAdoo & J. L. McAdoo (Eds.), *Black children: Social, educational, and parental environments* (pp. 159–173). Newbury Park, CA: Sage.

Rodgers, J. A. (1994, December). Spirituality: Being in context. *Spirituality Research Network Update.* Pittsburgh, PA: Institute for the Black Family.

Royse, D., & Turner, G. (1980). Strengths of Black families: A Black community's perspective. *Social Work, 25*(5), 407–409.

Sue, S. (1977). Community mental services to minority groups: Some optimism, some pessimism. *American Psychologist, 32,* 616–624.

Taylor, S. L. (1993). *In the spirit.* New York: Harper/Perennial.

Thomas, A., & Sillen, T. (1972). *Racism and psychiatry.* New York: Citadel Press.

Vanzant, I. (1983). *Value in the valley.* New York: Simon & Schuster.

Washington, H. A. (1994). Human guinea pigs. *Emerge, 7,* 24–35.

Williams, D. H. (1986). The epidemiology of mental illness in Afro-Americans. *Hospital and Community Psychiatry, 37*(1), 42–49.

Worthington, C. (1992). An examination of factors influencing the diagnosis and treatment of Black patients in the mental health systems. *Archives of Psychiatric Nursing, 6*(3), 195–204.

9

〜

Asian-Indian Americans

RAMASWAMY VISWANATHAN
MANOJ R. SHAH
ANWARUL AHAD

In this chapter we will discuss issues of importance in the treatment of anxiety disorders in Asian-Indian Americans. We will first present some background information on Asian-Indian culture. Then we will discuss the therapist–patient relationship and specific clinical conditions, with some case illustrations.

It should be recognized that for the major psychiatric disorders, there appear to be more similarities than differences across cultures in the nature of psychopathology and the core treatment principles, but there can be significant variations in the frequencies with which some symptoms appear across different cultures (Carstairs & Kapur, 1976; Jablensky, Sartorius, Gulbinat, & Ernberg, 1981; Sartorius, Jablensky, Gulbinat, & Ernberg, 1980). Cultural expectations can weigh heavily on the therapist–patient relationship and the implementation of treatment techniques. Culture can also influence the language of communication, determining which symptoms are readily communicated and which are not (Kleinman & Good, 1985). Different degrees of Americanization and socioeconomic factors also influence the presentation of the clinical condition and treatment. Even though cultural differences are discussed in this chapter, one should avoid the danger of stereotyping. Not all Asian-Indians are the same. There are substantial subcultural and individual differences. One should view the differences discussed here as guideposts that will sensitize the clinician to look for certain features, rather than as absolute rules.

BACKGROUND

Religion and Language

India has a long and rich cultural heritage. Hinduism is the dominant religion (80% of the population), Islam is the second major religion (15% of the population), and Buddhism, Christianity, Jainism, Sikhism, and Zoroastranism are the other major religions. The predominant language of India is Hindi, but not everyone is conversant with it as there are several other languages in India as well. People from the Indian subcontinent (whose major countries are India, Bangladesh, Pakistan, and Sri Lanka) share many cultural similarities, even if they belong to different religions and language groups. Pakistan and Bangladesh were part of India before the country was partitioned in 1947 when India gained independence from British rule. The principal religion and language of Pakistan are Islam and Urdu, of Bangladesh are Islam and Bengali, and of Sri Lanka are Buddhism and Sinhalese. English is used widely for higher education and business purposes in the Indian subcontinent, and educated people are fluent in English. There are also people of Indian origin in sizable numbers in Southeast Asia, Africa, the Caribbean, and other regions of the world.

Migration to the United States

Much of the Asian-Indian migration to the United States took place from the 1960s onward. According to the 1990 U.S. Census estimates, Asian Americans comprised 2.9% of the U.S. population, and Asian Indians comprised 11.2% of the Asian American population (Uba, 1994, pp. 2–3). Indians generally migrate to the United States for better material and educational opportunities and because of the aura associated with the West (Ananth & Ananth, 1996). Many initially have an idea of ultimately returning to India, but eventually opt to stay in the United States indefinitely. Once an individual migrates to the United States, other family members and relatives may also migrate through that individual's help. People generally maintain strong family ties to their extended family of origin in India.

Immigrants bring their own schema of the world based on their upbringing and culture. In their lifestyle, they often assimilate some of the cultural values of their new environment, while at the same time retaining their cultural identity and many of their original cultural values. Many Asian-Indian Americans develop dual identities, being "9-to-5" Americans in the workplace and Indians at home (Desai & Coelho, 1980).

Societal Differences

Clinicians need to be aware of some important ways in which Indian social structure differs from American society.

1. Indian society is more restrictive and rule bound, whereas American society is generally more permissive and open.
2. Indian society has a more rigid hierarchical structure. Obedience to elders and authority is expected. Gender roles are rigidly defined.
3. In the dimension of sociocentrism versus egocentrism, Indian culture is more sociocentric. Whereas in the United States personal autonomy and individuality are valued, in India conformity and collectivity are expected.
4. Privacy is not a priority. Boundaries within families or even between neighbors are porous. It is common for people to know what is happening in their neighbors' homes, and for people to be privy to many intimate details of their extended family members' lives.
5. Behavior is very much influenced by the concept of shame. One is always mindful of what the neighbors might think and is wary of bringing shame to the family.
6. Most marriages are arranged. The marriage is considered to be an alliance between two families, and the families play an important role in mate selection and the subsequent marital life. Public display of romantic affection is frowned upon.
7. There are extensive and complex extended family relationships and interactions. Many Indians used to live in joint families (brothers' families living together with their parents and unmarried sisters, under the authority of the eldest man), but this has been giving way to nuclear families (Srivastava, 1984). Many parents still live with their adult children.

Fundamental Values

There are some ingrained cultural values in the Asian-Indian individual that are relevant to treatment.

1. Family and society are considered more important than the individual. "Looking out for oneself " is considered selfish and shame-

ful. Sacrifice is highly valued. There is a constant, overriding sense of obligation to the family and the extended family.

2. The concept of the self is an extended self that includes the family. When an Indian thinks of his or her identity, it is blended with the identity of his or her family (Roland, 1988).

3. There is a considerable drive to belong to the group, to blend with the group, and to be part of the group. Separation and individuation are not promoted, and dependency or interdependency is fostered by society.

4. People often comfortably hold parallel, sometimes conflicting, belief systems and follow one or the other or both depending on the situation. For example, they may believe in karma or fate, or in predeterminism based on astrological positions at birth and how these match with one's spouse's astrological configuration. At the same time they may also believe in deliberate control of one's mental faculties and emotional response, and a person's capacity to overcome great odds and change the course of events.

5. Patience, self-control, self-discipline, and not yielding to passion are valued.

THERAPEUTIC ISSUES

Asians, in comparison to Caucasians, generally delay seeking help for psychiatric problems and tend to underutilize mental health services (Lam & Kavanagh, 1996). Most Asian-Indians go to the general practitioner for relief of mental health problems (Lloyd, 1992). There is a high expectation of the capability of the family doctor, and he or she is expected to solve all problems. Some patients may resort to alternative medical practices such as faith or spiritual healing or indigenous systems of medicine. Stigma and lack of awareness may also be barriers to seeing a mental health practitioner. General practitioners, internists, and family practitioners play an important role in destigmatizing mental health care and referring the patient. It is generally important for the mental health professional to explore and deal with the stigma issue as soon as a patient presents for treatment.

Contact Phase

In many instances it is a family member who initiates contact with the clinician's office. This should not necessarily be construed as lack of motivation on the part of the patient, as family members typically view it as their duty to take such an initiative, and the patient is assuming the culturally normative dependent patient role. The clinician should not be surprised if a call comes from a sibling, cousin, uncle, or aunt, or even a family friend, instead of the spouse of the patient. Relatives and friends are generally more closely involved with the health of the patient in Asian-Indian culture compared to Western culture. It is important to accept information from such people, thus acknowledging their importance, rather than saying outright that you would not like to talk to them and only the patient should make the call. Such a behavior might be viewed as arrogant and rude, as rejecting and insulting the helpful behavior, and may jeopardize the treatment by alienating a powerful family member. However, because making the patient take responsibility is an important component of psychotherapy, after acknowledging the caller, the clinician should also ask to speak to the patient over the telephone. A general statement such as "I would like to talk to the patient also before setting up an appointment" is quite appropriate.

The First Session

It can generally be expected that at least one family member and possibly more than one will accompany the patient for the first appointment. It is important to talk to the accompanying family members at some point in the session. Apart from acknowledging the accompanying person's helper role, one can also gain useful information from an external observer that complements the information given by the patient.

When you want to talk to the patient privately, you may encounter polite protest from the patient, who may say that it is not necessary: "I have nothing to hide from him or her. He or she can listen to whatever I have to say." This stems from devaluation of privacy and diffusion of self-boundaries. The therapist can say, "That might be so. But still I would like to talk to you alone. Later I can talk to him or her." It is important for the therapist to insist on privacy and assume responsibility for this request. Because it may be difficult for the patient to ask for privacy, the directive coming from the therapist absolves the patient of the responsibility of asking for it.

After you have explained to the patient privately your assessment of the problem and your recommendations, it is advisable again to meet conjointly with the family members and explain at least briefly, leaving out any information that you feel others need not know. This goes along with the patient's cultural value system and sets the stage for including the family in the treatment process, which is often crucial for treatment success. Family members can in fact be quite helpful in helping the patient with tasks such as graded *in vivo* exposure and reinforcing the therapist's message. Also many patients may need validation from the family that the therapist's opinion and recommendations are acceptable. It is also easier for the patient to implement the therapist's suggestions without a well-meaning family derailing them, which is less likely if the family has heard the suggestions directly from the therapist.

Psychoeducation

Indians are much more likely to accept biological explanations, such as "chemical imbalance" or "nerves," and conditioning and cognitive-behavioral explanations than psychodynamic explanations. At the same time they may expect too much of "will power," and patients and families need to be educated about learning and cognitive-behavioral principles and about the length and process of treatment.

Expectations of Treatment

Many Indians expect the treatment to be short term, with infrequent sessions. This generally does not create problems with pharmacotherapy and cognitive-behavioral therapy (CBT). In addition, doctors/clinicians are viewed as omnipotent. Many patients and families expect the doctor to provide a magical pill or vitamin that will quickly cure the condition.

Therapist–Patient Relationship

Many patients may want to gain personal knowledge of the therapist and may ask questions that may be construed as intrusive by the Western practitioner, such as "Where do you live? Are you married? Do you have children?" Many Indians get gratification in finding something in common between self and the other, and may try to establish some person or place known to both of you. Refusing to answer these questions may be viewed as rejection. The therapist may answer some of the questions to cement the therapeutic alliance, while deciding not to give specifics such as where one lives. Likewise patients may bring gifts, especially Asian-Indian artifacts. Refusing these gifts may be viewed as rejection.

There is an expectation of a paternalistic relationship, a submission to authority, and a desire to please the doctor. Although this may lead to carrying out of assignments, it may also in some cases lead to exaggerated reporting of positive response to therapeutic interventions, for example, anxiety reduction after relaxation training.

Interpretations may be taken as criticism, as not living up to the expectation of the authority figure (therapist), and may produce a sense of shame. The therapist must be attuned to this and deal with it sensitively.

Respect for authority also means that the patient and family may not question what the clinician says and may not voice disagreement even though they may, in fact, disagree or have some reservations. Therefore the clinician must be attentive to subtle nonverbal cues, and should also ask if the patients have any questions or disagreements.

Many Indians may approach the therapeutic relationship as a *guru–chela* (revered teacher–student) relationship (Neki, 1973). They hold the therapist in reverence and look forward to enlightening teachings that they can implement to solve their problems and to make changes within themselves, and, as such, they are very receptive to the therapist's statements.

Clinical Issues

Even though most Asian-Indian Americans are fluent in English, it is a second language for many. The patients' command of the English language may not be adequate to capture the essence of their symptoms. Some words have different meanings and connotations in Indian English as compared to American English; for example, "mad" means "psychotic," not "angry." It has been said that it is helpful to ask the patient if he or she dreams in English; if so, one can assume that the patient can authentically express his or her feelings through English (Jayakar, 1994).

Somatic presentations are more culturally and personally acceptable. Feeling weak or tired and describing various bodily sensations such as indigestion, burning sensations, and pain are more common than describing cognitive or emotional issues (Ananth, 1984; Bhatt, Tomenson, & Benjamin, 1989; Carstairs & Kapur, 1976; Chambers, Yeragani, & Keshavan, 1986; Gada, 1982; Keshavan, Yeragani, & Chambers, 1986; Rao, 1973; Saxena, Nepal, & Mohan, 1988; Sethi & Gupta, 1970; Srinivasan, Murthy, & Janakiramaiah, 1986; Teja, Narang, & Aggarwal, 1971). Among more educated and younger Indians, there may be less tendency to somatize (Ullrich, 1993). Fears of sudden death and illness are common among Indian phobic patients (Chambers et al., 1986; Keshavan et al., 1986).

Indian patients with anxiety disorders often feel a sense of shame and inadequacy. They believe that one should be able to "psyche oneself out." A therapist can use this belief as the seed for CBT. At the same time one can deal with the sense of shame through psychoeducation and through cognitive therapy (e.g., pointing out overgeneralizations, perfectionism, selective attention, arbitrary inference, etc.).

Indians' philosophical system, which puts a great emphasis on deliberate control of mental faculties and self-discipline, can be harnessed in the service of CBT. Indian patients and families are very receptive to relaxation training, breathing control, changing one's attitudes toward problems and events, and changing how one looks at the situation.

Indians have an age-old tradition of *pranayama*, which involves a particular form of rhythmic breathing while chanting some sacred sounds (Ornish, 1990, pp. 164–171). Many believe in the mental changes produced by it. So they will enthusiastically adopt the breathing retraining taught by many behavioral practitioners. Yoga and meditation are other time-honored systems designed to bring about mental and physical health (Chopra, 1987; Ornish, 1990, pp. 139–146, 234–251; Singh, 1986). In fact, if the therapist is familiar with these systems, he may substitute them for progressive relaxation training and other common behavioral interventions (Wolpe, 1990, pp. 195–196).

The patient may not see any need to reveal his inner feelings. This may be due to a cultural tendency to discourage open expression of feelings, as well as due to the expectation that the clinician has an almost magical ability to figure out and correct problems without much help from the patient.

In general, Indians are more interested in symptom reduction than in resolving unconscious conflicts (Ananth, 1984). Indeed, talking ill of one's parents or childhood upbringing is not culturally acceptable. Motherhood is highly valued for its sacrifices, and hence to talk about negative aspects of one's mother, even in the context of an overall positive opinion, is almost sacrilegious.

The influence of the extended family structure can be both problematic and helpful. On one hand, problems such as dissatisfaction with in-laws, interference by grandparents in child care, contradictory communications, disharmonious sibling interactions, marital conflict, and lack of cooperation and support from relatives can provoke significant anxiety in many patients (Rao, Channabasavanna, & Parthasarathy, 1984). Despite this, many patients may be reluctant to work on questioning the authority structure of the family. On the other hand, family involvement and support often facilitate therapeutic interventions such as *in vivo* exposure assignments and relaxation procedures (Mehta & Ochaney, 1987).

Religion or spiritual faith plays an important role in many patients' lives, and the clinician should help the patient make constructive use of it. Patients may also be using indigenous remedies such as herbal medicines or talismans. In the early phase of the treatment, it is not advisable for the therapist to criticize such remedies unless they are harmful or have adverse interactions with prescription medications (see Chapter 10).

Gender Issues

Gender roles in Indian society are well defined. The husband is the master of the home. Women are expected to be dependent on the men. Many Indian women were brought up to be docile and subservient to their husbands and in-laws, and not to express negative feelings (Jayakar, 1994). Although these features are changing even in Indian society, they still influence the dynamics of many women. Some women may not talk freely to a male therapist. It is important to include the husband in the treatment process so as to prevent sabotage and to facilitate changes. Many Indian women manage to be Western at work and Indian at home (Jayakar, 1994). When a husband has panic disorder with agoraphobia, it can create considerable strain in the marital relationship. The wife has the difficult task of doing traditional male chores such as driving, while at the same time not bruising the male ego. Out of a sense of shame, male agoraphobic patients tend to hide their fear from others. On the other hand, agoraphobia in women is much more easily tolerated by the culture as it is congruent with the traditional woman's role of dependence on others.

It should be noted that India has had some women in leadership positions such as a prime minister, state governors, and state chief ministers. There are a considerable number of women Indian physicians and other professionals, both in India and in the United States. The society has two coexisting value systems, one suppressing women, and the other revering them and allowing them accomplishments outside the home. This knowledge is important for therapists treating Indian women who have anxieties that interfere with career success. Therapists doing assertiveness training with Indian women should take care to promote assertiveness in such a way that it improves self-esteem and functioning without making the woman a cultural misfit.

Culture-Bound Syndromes

Koro, a culture-bound syndrome reported in Indians and other Asians, can be considered an acute anxiety state, somatoform disorder, depersonalization, or psychosis (Bernstein & Gaw, 1990; Griffith & Gonzalez, 1994; Yap, 1965). In Malay, *koro* means the head of a turtle; its symbolism as glans penis probably gave rise to the name of the syndrome (Yap, 1965). *Koro*, which can appear sporadically or occasionally in miniepidemics, includes an intense fear that the penis is shrinking or disappearing into the abdomen, with associated features of guilt and shame about nocturnal emission, masturbation, or other sexual activity. The shrinking of the penis or its disappearance into the abdomen is thought to be punishment for sins committed. This condition responds to psychotherapy and tranquilizers (Yap, 1965).

Dhat syndrome is a culture-bound sex neurosis found in the Indian subcontinent (Chadda & Ahuja, 1990). Patients believe that they are losing semen (*dhat*) in their urine and that this leads to depletion of physical and mental energy. They present with multiple somatic complaints along with feelings of physical and mental exhaustion that they attribute to the passage of semen in their urine. Many cases are associated with depression or anxiety disorders (Chadda & Ahuja, 1990). Many patients improve with sexual counseling and treatment of associated anxiety disorder or depression (Behere & Natraj, 1984).

Other Culture-Sensitive Anxiety Disorders

Although the patient's culture pervades any clinical situation, there are some disorders where the influence of culture can be quite strong. The following are some examples.

Obsessive–Compulsive Disorder

Obsessive–compulsive disorder is often influenced by religious and cultural context, more so than many other disorders. Hinduism has many rituals, and there is great variability among Indians in the extent to which these rituals are practiced. Many obsessive–compulsive disorder rituals may not be recognized as such by the society, and the society may accommodate the individual's rituals as spiritual or religious. Usually it takes considerable impairment and long duration before an individual is brought to clinical attention. On the other hand, to a clinician not conversant with the culture, the culturally influenced obsessions and rituals may appear to be psychotic. Clinicians treating obsessive–compulsive disorder patients should educate themselves

about the relevant cultural and religious issues, through discussions
with the patient and the family and with professionals familiar with
the particular culture. The following case is an example of these issues.

A professional in his 40s sought help for obsessions and compulsions
that were present since adolescence, but had become much worse in
the past few years. The predominant obsessions concerned whether
he had desecrated God; he feared punishment for it. In the mornings,
when he stepped out of his home, he would wonder if he should step
on the ground, because God was everywhere, and whether if he
stepped on the ground, it would mean he was stepping on God. He
would try to take the step back. Still he worried if God would punish
him for this transgression. If he stepped forward again, the same
doubts would bother him, and again he would step back. He would
spend considerable time obsessing about it, repeatedly stepping back
and forth, and praying as a way of warding off punishment. Eventually he would move forward, but still with considerable obsessive
ruminations. He was often late going to work and to many appointments because of this. He had difficulty in even leaving the therapist's
office after a session was over. If he had to close a door, he was
concerned that he might have hit God (as God is everywhere), and he
would repeatedly open and close the door. He could not drive because
of his obsessions about hitting God. He spent considerable time
praying to God to atone for his desecration of God. At times he felt,
"If I were dead, I would get freedom from this tyranny." He was also
concerned that his child had begun copying his repeated stepping
back and forth.

The patient had tried pharmacological treatment with another
clinician in the past, but it was not helpful. In his adolescence and
young adulthood, he used to obsess about whether he had desecrated
Goddess Saraswathi (Goddess of Education in Hinduism) and
whether she would punish him by making him forget what he had
learned and by making him fail his examinations. The obsessive–compulsive disorder did interfere with his examination performance, and
he used to run away from home out of shame when he did not do as
well as he could have done. The patient never told his family about
his obsessive–compulsive disorder.

Clinicians should be aware that in Hinduism it is sacrilegious to
wear footwear in places of worship, and for the foot to come in contact
with sacred objects, including books (which are treated as manifestations of Goddess Saraswathi). At a different philosophical level, one
school of Hinduism believes not only that God is everywhere, but that
everything in this world is made of God's divine substance (also
called *brahman*), that all objects in this universe are manifestations of
God. The patient's psychotherapy took these aspects into account and

consisted of psychoeducational measures including socratic questioning of his assumptions. It was pointed out to him that which rule one
follows depends on the context. Certain areas are designated by
society as sacred, as symbols of God, and the rules of not stepping on
apply only to these symbols, just like designating a piece of cloth as
a national flag, a symbol of a nation, and saluting it; stepping on this
piece of cloth is considered sacrilegious, whereas one can step on
other pieces of cloth, and, of course, on the ground of the nation itself.
The patient was gradually led to see that if God designed this world
and if God was everywhere, then it would be safe to assume that His
intent was to allow us to walk on some aspects of Him; that he was
not following Hinduism, but his own idiosyncratic notion of it, as,
historically, Hindu religious figures had no qualms about stepping on
the ground. *In vivo* prolonged exposure with response prevention was
also carried out (stepping forward with one foot and holding that
position for a long time without withdrawing the foot). In addition,
imaginal flooding about God's anger at him for stepping on Him
during his regular walking was utilized.

Social Phobias and Anxiety

Social phobias and anxiety are accentuated by submissiveness, unas-
sertiveness, and deference to others, and by being in an alien culture.
Many Asian-Indians are brought up with the notion that one should
not speak up, should be cognizant of the power hierarchy, and should
avoid sustained eye contact. In American society, which prizes assertiveness and where social boundaries are not as rigid, these traits may
become shortcomings. Some patients are also acutely sensitive to
looking different than the dominant ethnic groups. The therapist
should help patients take pride in their own identity, while at the same
time respecting other cultures, and assimilating with the American
culture. Assertiveness training and communication skills training are
found to be helpful by many socially anxious patients.

A 26-year-old Asian-Indian man felt isolated at work. He would eat
his lunch alone, as he was afraid that others would laugh at his ethnic
food; he was also afraid that he would be tongue-tied and not be able
to carry on conversations with others. He had low self-esteem and felt
that others would look down on him and not respect him because of
his different culture and ethnicity. He would panic if he had to speak
or present something at meetings. He did not get promoted because
of these anxieties. The patient was encouraged to see that, if he
accepted himself, then perhaps others would accept him. Through
cognitive therapy he was made to question some of the assumptions

he was making about himself and others and to appreciate the role of self-fulfilling prophecies. He received assertiveness training, including behavior rehearsal and anxiety-reduction procedures.

Adjustment Reaction with Anxiety

Adjustment reaction with anxiety is common among newly arrived immigrants. Unfamiliarity with the conversational language (including slang) and being unaccustomed to new behavior patterns can add to the sense of insecurity.

> A professional who had recently migrated to the United States from India began experiencing anxiety attacks, bordering on panic, whenever he had to drive. He had driven a car in India without any difficulty. However, in a big city in the United States, some drivers had used abusive language and gestures to ridicule his slow (in their opinion) driving responses. He felt insulted and belittled by people who he felt were less educated and in a "lower position" than he was. Through psychoeducation and acculturation he quickly learned not to let himself be bothered too much by such remarks, and his driving anxiety disappeared.

Sexual Anxiety

Even though India is known as the land of Kamasutra, Indian society is in actuality much more sexually repressive than Western societies. Because most marriages are arranged, premarital sex is not condoned by society. There is no sex education in school, and many people are ignorant or ill informed about the physiological and psychological aspects of human sexuality. When a newly married couple tries to have sexual intercourse for the first time in their lives, if the man cannot successfully maintain an erection for whatever reason, it is often viewed as a personal defect, engendering performance anxiety. Men view themselves as "impotent" instead of trying to understand the causes of erectile failure. Women also can have various anxieties that interfere with the enjoyment of sexual intercourse. If the couple comes for treatment early, most of these problems can be solved by simple educational measures and reassurance. In light of the cultural message of sexual repression, it can be therapeutic for the couple to get permission from an authority figure (the clinician) that it is all right for the couple to enjoy sex. The clinician can also stress the importance of communicating their needs to each other. The clinician may find that many patients become uncomfortable when sexuality is discussed and should be sensitive to this issue (Ananth, 1984).

> An Asian-Indian professional man married an Asian-Indian woman in the United States through an arranged marriage. The first time the couple tried sexual intercourse, the husband could not penetrate the wife because of the couple's anxiety and inexperience. The husband became very worried about his potency, and the performance anxiety led to failure in further attempts. The husband also began worrying that soon their families would suspect or find out about his sexual problem, and it would bring shame to him and his family. This sent the husband into a panic state and resulted in an emergency psychiatric consultation. A single conjoint session with the husband and wife that involved education, reassurance, and opening up communication resulted in resolution of the problem. The couple has now been happily married for several years, and they have four children.

Test Anxiety

Test anxiety is clinically a much more serious situation for Indians than for non-Asians (Chambers et al., 1986). Because there are many Indian students in the United States, therapists should be sensitive to this issue. Asian American parents in general put greater pressure on their children for academic achievement than do European Americans (Uba, 1994, pp. 44–46). Examination failure is considered shameful by many middle-class Indians, not only to the individual, but to the family as well, and in some cases, it may lead to suicide. Even if one passed the examination with good grades, if one did not measure up to the highest standards, this can lead to considerable dysphoria and feelings of failure. It is of interest that an early report of flooding therapy (Malleson, 1959) concerned the treatment of an Indian student who was terribly afraid of examinations. The imagined consequences of failure were derision from colleagues in India, disappointment from family, and his wife and mother being in tears.

Somatization

Because expression or acknowledgment of negative affect toward family members is unacceptable, anxiety and depression are often expressed through somatization. Somatic symptoms such as weakness, tiredness, dizziness, chest pains, choking sensation, feeling of pressure in the neck, and tingling sensations in various parts of the body, and hypochondriasis, are often the ticket to get help for psychological stress. There can be more dramatic conversion symptom presentations, such as pseudoepileptic attacks and paralysis.

A woman developed paralysis of her legs after her husband received a kidney transplant from his sister. It appeared to have been due to her anxiety that her husband's indebtedness to his sister would prevent him from defending his wife against the sister-in-law's verbal attacks. Exploration of this changed family dynamic and reassurance from the husband that he would continue to defend his wife led to amelioration of the wife's symptoms.

A man developed an intense fear of heart attack, after a mild elevation in blood pressure was discovered during one of his visits to his doctor. He gave a history of having dated a woman in India after they were engaged to each other for arranged marriage. The engagement was called off by his family because of conflict between the two families, even though he and the woman liked each other, and he did not assert himself. He, as well as the woman, subsequently got married to other people and had happy marriages. The diagnosis of high blood pressure activated fears of punishment by God or some supernatural force for his bringing shame to this woman by dating her but not marrying her. Alleviation of guilt and correction of magical thinking through CBT helped resolve his fear.

An Indian female physician was experiencing attacks of chest pain, dizziness, sweating, and fear that she might pass out or die, lasting about half an hour. The attacks were precipitated when she was involved in an argument, or if she was experiencing anger and not expressing it. She had had a few medical emergency room visits and an extensive medical workup that did not reveal any abnormalities. She improved with CBT, including anxiety-reduction techniques, problem solving, and coping more adaptively with her anger.

Agoraphobia without Panic

Because of the dependency fostered in women by the Indian society, agoraphobia without panic disorder is apparently more common among Indian women in the United States compared to American-born women. The condition responds favorably to therapist-guided graded *in vivo* exposure coupled with social skills training. But at times, system dynamics can complicate the treatment.

A married Indian woman who was unassertive and agoraphobic was helped to overcome her phobia and become more assertive through behavior therapy. As she made progress, her husband, who denied any prior history of psychiatric problems, became acutely depressed. It became apparent that his self-esteem was partly based on his wife's dependency on him. Fortunately, the husband agreed to seek psychotherapy for his problems.

Children and Adolescents

Children do not grow up in a vacuum. They cannot be understood apart from the historical, geographical, and socioeconomic characteristics of the area in which they develop. The children we see are members not only of families but also of wider groups, whose training patterns affect them a good deal. We need to be aware of these cultural patterns; only then will we be able to understand the child's own functioning and that of his or her family in an adequate way (Looff, 1979).

Immigrant children experience some conflicts between the schema of their upbringing and the schema of the host culture, and they strive for resolution and compromise. What may be considered pathological in Western society may not apply if the therapist is aware of the practices among immigrants from the Indian subcontinent. For example, children sleep in the parents' bedroom or even in the parental bed to an extended (compared to American children) age of 2 or 3 years. When the parents then try to get the child out of their bedroom, it may lead to anxiety, manifested in the form of sleep difficulties, delayed sleep, or nightmares, or the child may resist going to his or her bedroom. Independence and individuation are not fostered in many homes, and this may lead to separation anxiety disorder or school phobia when the child is ready to be placed in a nursery school, or may manifest as an anxiety disorder when the person enters an out-of-town college.

> A 17-year-old Indian girl presented with symptoms of difficulty with breathing, inability to sleep due to a sense of suffocation, and having to keep the windows in her bedroom open even during the winter months. When her anxieties about going away to an out-of-town college were explored and resolved, the above symptoms disappeared.

Another specific cultural practice that may be seen by the clinician is that some parents send away their young children to India. At a young age, when both parents are studying or working, instead of entrusting the care of the child to a babysitter or nanny, or to day care, the child may be sent to India to be raised by grandparents. Later, when the child returns to the United States at a convenient time for the parents, various anxiety-related symptoms may surface. These may take the form of not interacting with the parents, withdrawal, sleep difficulties, enuresis, and communication difficulties. The communication difficulties may take the form of selective mutism. Adjustment problems in school may also occur.

> A 4½-year-old Indian boy was brought for psychiatric evaluation due to temper tantrums, aggressive behavior, and using bad language. He also had difficulties falling asleep, nightmares, and secondary functional enuresis. The psychosocial history revealed that he was born in New York and sent to India at age 6 months, was reared by grandparents, and had returned to New York at age 4 years to rejoin his parents. An extensive medical evaluation for enuresis was avoided by knowing the cultural background of this child. The parents were reassured that this was an adjustment reaction. The child improved after several months of therapy.

Indian children are generally not referred for specific phobias. For example, Hackett, Hackett, and Taylor (1991), found that phobias were common among Gujarati (an Indian community) children in England, but aroused no parental concern. As a result, psychiatric service was not sought for these disorders. Social phobias and selective mutism are also common, particularly in view of the cultural mandate to make one's own needs subservient to the needs of the others, and the discouragement of asserting oneself. Performance anxiety in a variety of situations, including performing in a concert or speaking publicly are seen frequently.

Obsessive–compulsive disorder does interfere with daily functioning, not only of the child but also of the family, and children of Asian-Indian origin with this disorder do come to the attention of the mental health professionals. As noted before, the rituals can be influenced by cultural or religious beliefs.

> A 14-year-old boy developed a compulsion to mumble a phrase after shaking his head from side to side. Apparently he was experiencing sexual thoughts, which were considered taboo by his cultural upbringing. He would shake his head to ward off these thoughts and then mumble a prayer in his native language asking for forgiveness. To an onlooker who did not understand the language and did not know the reasoning, the behavior appeared psychotic.

The fear of failure in an examination with the concomitant bringing of shame on the family leads to a significant degree of anxiety, and many children thus come to the attention of the mental health professionals—more so in their pubertal and adolescent years. If untreated, the risk of suicide in such cases is significant, as noted above.

> Two brothers ran away from school because they had grades that were not up to their father's expectations. They expressed fear that their father would hit them if they did poorly in school. He also would get angry and hit them if the teacher wrote any negative comments about their behavior, as he believed that it reflected badly on the family name. He did not listen to the children's side of the story, claiming the teacher was always right. The children were depressed, and the older son had even thought of suicide. The mother, who was seen separately, reluctantly confirmed the story. The father was then seen alone, and later along with his wife and children. A behavior modification program for the children with rewards and acceptable punishments was worked out, to the satisfaction of both the parents and the children.

During the process of evaluating a child, an adequate history from the parents first needs to be obtained, as many parents come with the expectation that the therapist, who is seen as an almost divine, all-knowing authority figure, will have all the answers. Second, there is a tendency to report only a few symptoms so that the therapist does not look upon the family negatively. Third, the family may feel a need to minimize the condition, as there is a belief that if there are more symptoms, the child is sicker. As noted previously, there is an added issue of stigma attached to consulting a mental health professional. There is also the belief that any emotional illness is equivalent to being "crazy." Psychoeducation of the parents is the first step in the treatment and management of these children. Besides the parents, if there are other significant adults, they also need to be seen and their cooperation obtained. Issues of confidentiality have to be carefully addressed, particularly when the patient is an adolescent who has grown up in the United States. Behavior modification has to be approached with caution as the parents expect the child to conform rather than their having to reward a child for positive behavior (Uba, 1994, p. 48). Behavior modification that involves rewards are seen as an assault on the authority status of the parent in addition to being a bribe to the child. The families also expect a quick cure, and this expectation has to be addressed.

Psychopharmacology

Indians, like other Asians, generally appear to need lower doses of psychotropic medications such as benzodiazepines, antidepressants, and antipsychotics, compared to Western patients (Griffith & Gonzalez, 1994; Yamamoto & Lin, 1995). This may be due to slower metabolism or greater sensitivity. Clinically, it has been our experience that Indian patients generally accept medications much more readily compared to many Caucasian anxiety disorder patients and are generally not afraid of medications. In fact, patients often ask for a "strong" medication. The family also gets involved with medication issues.

SUMMARY

There are some important differences between the societal structures and fundamental values of Asian-Indian and American cultures. Hence there is a need on the part of the "clinician to move beyond the limitations of traditional assessment, diagnostic and treatment approaches and learn how to determine the impact of cultural differences and acculturation issues" (Canino & Spurlock, 1994, front inside cover) in planning therapy for people from the Indian subcontinent. The clinician should be sensitive to the cultural influence on the therapist–patient relationship, the role of the family, some culture-specific clinical situations, and some indigent therapeutic practices. At the same time, one should avoid the pitfall of stereotyping. Not all Indians are the same, and there are substantial subcultural and individual differences. Clinicians treating Asian-Indian patients will find it to be an enriching and rewarding experience.

REFERENCES

Ananth, J. (1984). Treatment of immigrant Indian patients. *Canadian Journal of Psychiatry, 29,* 490–493.

Ananth, J., & Ananth, K. (1996). *East Indian immigrants to the United States: Life cycle issues and adjustment.* East Meadow, NY: Indo-American Psychiatric Association.

Behere, P. B., & Natraj, G. S. (1984). Dhat syndrome: The phenomenology of a culture bound sex neurosis of the Orient. *Indian Journal of Psychiatry, 26,* 76–78.

Bernstein, R. L., & Gaw, A. C. (1990). Koro: Proposed classification for DSM-IV. *American Journal of Psychiatry, 147,* 1670–1674.

Bhatt, A., Tomenson, B., & Benjamin, S. (1989). Transcultural patterns of somatization in primary care: A preliminary report. *Journal of Psychosomatic Research, 33,* 671–680.

Canino, I. A., & Spurlock, J. (1994). *Culturally diverse children and adolescents: Assessment, diagnosis and treatment.* New York: Guilford Press.

Carstairs, G. M., & Kapur, G. L. (1976). *Great universe of Kota.* London: Hogarth Press.

Chadda, R. K., & Ahuja, N. (1990). Dhat syndrome: A sex neurosis of the Indian subcontinent. *British Journal of Psychiatry, 156,* 577–579.

Chambers, J., Yeragani, V. K., & Keshavan, M. S. (1986). Phobias in India and the United Kingdom. *Acta Psychiatrica Scandinavica, 74,* 388–391.

Chopra, D. (1987). *Creating health: Beyond prevention, toward perfection.* Boston: Houghton Miffin.

Desai, P., & Coelho, G. (1980). Indian immigrants in America: Some cultural aspects of psychological adaptation. In P. Saran & E. Eames (Eds.), *The new ethnics: Asian Indians in the United States* (pp. 369–386). New York: Praeger.

Gada, M. T. (1982). A cross cultural study of symptomatology of depression: Eastern versus Western patients. *International Journal of Social Psychiatry, 28,* 195–202.

Griffith, E. E. H., & Gonzalez, C. A. (1994). Essentials of cultural psychiatry. In R. E. Hales, S. C. Yudofsky, & J. A. Talbott (Eds.), *American Psychiatric Association textbook of psychiatry* (2nd ed., pp. 1379–1401). Washington, DC: American Psychiatric Press.

Hackett, L., Hackett, R., & Taylor, D. C. (1991). Psychological disturbance and its association in the children of the Gujarati community. *Journal of Child Psychology and Psychiatry, 32,* 851–856.

Jablensky, A., Sartorius, N., Gulbinat, W., & Ernberg, G. (1981). Characteristics of depressive patients contacting psychiatric services in four cultures. *Acta Psychiatrica Scandinavica, 63,* 367–383.

Jayakar, K. (1994). Women of the Indian subcontinent. In L. Comas-Díaz & B. Greene (Eds.), *Women of color: Integrating ethnic and gender identities in psychotherapy* (pp. 161–181). New York: Guilford Press.

Keshavan, M. S., Yeragani, V. K., & Chambers J. (1986). Phobic neuroses in India: A cross-cultural comparison [Letter to editor]. *British Journal of Psychiatry, 148,* 341–342.

Kleinman, A., & Good, B. (Eds.). (1985). *Culture and depression: Studies in the anthropology and cross-cultural psychiatry of affect and disorder.* Berkeley, CA: University of California Press.

Lam, A. P., & Kavanagh, D. J. (1996). Help seeking by immigrant Indochinese psychiatric patients in Sydney, Australia. *Psychiatric Services, 47,* 993–995.

Lloyd, K. (1992). Ethnicity, primary care and non-psychotic disorders. *International Review of Psychiatry, 4,* 257–265.

Looff, D. (1979). Sociocultural factors in etiology. In J. D. Noshpitz (Ed.), *Basic handbook of child psychiatry* (Vol. 2, pp. 87–89). New York: Basic Books.

Malleson, N. (1959). Panic and phobia. *Lancet, 1,* 225–227.

Mehta, M., & Ochaney, M. (1987). Assessing the efficacy of home practice relaxation procedure. *Journal of Personality and Clinical Studies, 3,* 145–147.

Neki, J. S. (1973). Guru–chela relationship. *American Journal of Orthopsychiatry, 43,* 755–766.

Ornish, D. (1990). *Dr. Dean Ornish's program for reversing heart disease.* New York: Ballantine Books.

Rao, A. (1973). Depression: A psychiatric analysis of thirty cases. *Indian Journal of Psychiatry, 15,* 231–236.

Rao, V. N., Channabasavanna, S. M., & Parthasarathy, R. (1984). Anxiety provoking situations in Indian families. *International Journal of Social Psychiatry, 30,* 218–221.

Roland, A. (1988). *In search of self in India and Japan: Toward a cross-cultural psychology.* Princeton, NJ: Princeton University Press.

Sartorius, N., Jablensky, A., Gulbinat, W., & Ernberg, G. (1980). WHO collaborative study: Assessment of depressive disorders. *Psychological Medicine, 10,* 743–749.

Saxena, S., Nepal, M. K., & Mohan, D. (1988). DSM-III Axis 1 diagnoses of Indian psychiatric patients with somatic symptoms. *American Journal of Psychiatry, 145,* 1023–1024.

Sethi, B., & Gupta, S. (1970). An epidemiological and cultural study of depression. *Indian Journal of Psychiatry, 12,* 13–22.

Singh, R. H. (1986). Evaluation of some Indian traditional methods of promotion of mental health. *Activitas Nervosa Superior, 28,* 67–69.

Srinivasan, K., Murthy, R. S., & Janakiramaiah, N. (1986). A nosological study of patients presenting with somatic complaints. *Acta Psychiatrica Scandinavica, 73,* 1–5.

Srivastava, R. K. (1984). Family structure, manifest anxiety and disclosure of self among urban boys. *Psychological Studies, 29,* 169–171.

Teja, J. S., Narang, R. L., & Aggarwal, A. K. (1971). Depression across cultures. *British Journal of Psychiatry, 119,* 253–260.

Uba, L. (1994). *Asian Americans: Personality patterns, identity, and mental health.* New York: Guilford Press.

Ullrich, H. E. (1993). Cultural shaping and illness: A longitudinal perspective on apparent depression. *Journal of Nervous and Mental Disease, 181,* 647–649.

Wolpe, J. (1990). *The practice of behavior therapy* (4th ed.). New York: Pergamon Press.

Yamamoto, J., & Lin, K.-M., (1995). Psychopharmacology, ethnicity, and culture. In J. M. Oldham & M. B. Riba (Eds.), *American Psychiatric Press review of psychiatry* (Vol. 14, pp. 529–541). Washington, DC: American Psychiatric Press.

Yap, P. M. (1965). Koro: A culture-bound depersonalization syndrome. *British Journal of Psychiatry, 111,* 43–50.

III

~

SPECIAL TOPICS

10

Psychopharmacology and Ethnicity

IRA M. LESSER
MICHAEL SMITH
RUSSELL E. POLAND
KEH-MING LIN

Ethnicity and culture exert powerful influences on the effects of a wide array of medications, including the majority of psychotropics (Kalow, 1991, 1992). Numerous reports in the past four decades have indicated that substantial cross-ethnic differences exist in the dosage requirement and side effect profiles of various psychotropic medications. Advances in the fields of pharmacokinetics, pharmacodynamics, and pharmaco-genetics have begun to shed light on some of the mechanisms that may be responsible for these differences (Kalow, 1992; Lesser, Lin, & Poland, 1994; Lin & Poland, 1995). In comparison, less information is available regarding the influence of factors more immediately mediated by culture, but integral to the process of taking medications, such as treatment compliance, placebo effect, and physicians' biases. In the treatment of patients with anxiety disorders, where medications are often combined with a variety of psychotherapeutic interventions, attention must be given both to the biological factors associated with pharmacological treatment and to the more culturally mediated responses to taking medications.

Clinically, the importance of culture and ethnicity in health care is increasingly apparent, considering the rapid diversification of the population in all metropolitan areas of the world. Because of the large-scale population shifts and the rapid pace of intercontinental transportation and migration, most psychiatrists can no longer, nor should they, limit their practice to culturally or ethnically homogeneous groups. Patients' divergent beliefs, expectations, dietary practices, and genetic constitutions must be taken into consideration in psychopharmacotherapy. This is part of the reason that the National Institutes of Health and the Food and Drug Administration have started to pay attention to ethnicity as a factor in the research activities that fall under their aegis. This chapter will focus on these aspects of the interface between pharmacology and ethnicity in general, while at the same time discussing areas specific to anxiety disorders.

Beginning almost four decades ago, the introduction of various psychotropics, now mainstays of treating anxiety disorders, led to revolutionary changes in the practice of psychiatry. Although originally developed in Western Europe and North America, they were quickly introduced and extensively utilized for the treatment of psychiatric patients in countries and societies with divergent racial/ethnic backgrounds, socioeconomic conditions, and cultural traditions. At the same time, with immigration and increased ease and flexibility in movements around the globe, societies within a given country have become more heterogeneous, requiring clinicians to understand not only how illness may present differently across ethnicities or cultures, but how treatment modalities and side effects may, likewise, be different.

Despite an apparent "universal" utility and efficacy of psychopharmacotherapeutic agents, there have been many reports of crossnational and cross-cultural variations in dosing practices and side effect profiles. Most of the reports of ethnic differences in psychotropics have contrasted Caucasians with non-Caucasians, particularly Asians, African Americans, and Hispanics, although virtually no attention has been given to Native Americans (Mendoza, Smith, Poland, Lin, & Strickland, 1991). This chapter will start with an outline of mechanisms governing drug responses. With this as background, the influence of ethnicity and culture on various aspects of drug response will be systematically presented. Finally, the clinical and research implications of these findings, as well as future research directions, will be discussed.

MECHANISMS AFFECTING DRUG METABOLISM AND ACTION

Numerous factors are involved in determining how an individual responds to a particular medication. These factors not only vary among individuals, but often are influenced significantly by ethnicity and cultural factors. Mechanisms responsible for cross-ethnic differences in drug response are similar to those that determine interindividual variability in the dose range and side effect profiles, and can be classified into three major categories: pharmacokinetics, pharmacodynamics, and sociocultural factors (Greenblatt, 1993).

The "biological" effects of pharmacological agents are determined by pharmacokinetic and pharmacodynamic processes. Simply stated, as it applies to humans, pharmacokinetics is the study of how the body affects the fate and distribution of a drug, whereas pharmacodynamics deals with how the drug affects the body. The pharmacokinetics of most drugs are determined by four basic processes: absorption, distribution, metabolism, and excretion (Greenblatt, 1993; Preskorn, 1993). Of these, metabolism has been identified as most likely to contribute to interindividual and cross-ethnic variations (Kalow, 1993; Lin, Poland, & Nakasaki, 1993).

Drugs and other foreign substances are metabolized by a number of enzymes whose activities vary substantially across individuals and ethnic groups. In recent years, a large number of drug-metabolizing enzymes, as well as the genes responsible for encoding these enzymes, have been identified and characterized. Many of these enzymes and their genes are present in two or more distinct forms within a given population, a condition known as "polymorphism." Often, multiple forms of mutations lead to inactivation or reduced activity of the enzymes (Kalow, 1992). Substantial ethnic variations exist in the frequency of these gene mutations (genotypes) and the enzyme activity (phenotypes) of many of these polymorphic drug-metabolizing enzymes. Because these enzymes are responsible for the metabolism of many of the medications commonly used in clinical settings, variations in their activity will be reflected in significant differences in the pharmacokinetics of the drug, possibly resulting in variations in therapeutic dose ranges and side effect profiles.

Ethnicity, Pharmacokinetics, and Pharmacogenetics

From a historical perspective, one of the most striking examples highlighting the interplay of genetics and drug response occurred during

World War II, when American soldiers fighting in the Pacific theater were routinely given the drug primaquine for the prevention of malaria. Subsequently, a large number of soldiers, almost exclusively of African American descent, developed severe hemolytic anemia. Investigations led to the discovery in these men of an inborn deficiency of the enzyme glucose-6-phosphate dehydrogenase. It was discovered that the absence of this enzyme in a person exposed to a variety of substances, including primaquine, would result in the development of hemolytic anemia (Kalow, 1990, 1992).

The first antituberculosis medication, isoniazid, was introduced in 1952. Soon, it was observed that the side effect profiles of this medication were quite different in Asians and Caucasians. Whereas Asians manifested a higher rate of liver disease (obstructive hepatitis), Caucasians were more likely to develop neurological symptoms (peripheral neuritis). This observation led to the finding of a differential rate of acetylation, a step in the elimination of isoniazid, between members of these ethnic groups. Although the technology was not available at the time, molecular biological techniques subsequently have identified specific loci of point mutations among subjects from different ethnic groups, which are responsible for slow acetylation (Weber, 1987).

A third example of particular interest because of the high comorbidity of anxiety disorders and alcohol abuse is the "flushing response" in a large number of Asians when exposed to alcohol (Argawal & Goedde, 1990; Yoshida, 1993). First reported by Wolff (1972) among Asian immigrants residing in the United States, this condition was subsequently found to exist in more than 50% of Eastern Asians including Chinese, Japanese, Koreans, and Vietnamese. Similarly, high percentages of "flushing response" were reported among Highland Central and South American Indians (Yoshida, 1993). Typical "flushers" report rapid facial flushing, dizziness, palpitations, nausea, and other uncomfortable symptoms after ingesting even a very small amount of an alcoholic beverage. As in the examples given above, the mechanisms underlying this clinical observation awaited advances in technology. It is now known that in the metabolism of alcohol, a genetically determined deficiency of the enzyme aldehyde dehydrogenase results in the rapid accumulation of acetaldehyde, which is highly toxic and capable of inducing all the symptoms listed above. In fact, the therapeutic basis of disulfiram (Antabuse) is based on its ability to inhibit the activities of acetaldehyde dehydrogenase.

As mentioned above, the contribution that genetics makes to a large number of drug-metabolizing enzymes is well established. The activities of many of these enzymes, similar to the examples given above, show substantial cross-ethnic differences. Among these, the cytochrome P450 enzyme system has received the most attention, particularly because this system clearly relates to clinical issues and the use of psychotropic medications (DeVane, 1994; Gonzalez, 1989, 1992; Kalow, 1991, 1992; Lin & Poland, 1995; Nemeroff, DeVane, & Pollock, 1996; Pollock, 1994; Riesenman, 1995).

Ethnicity and Pharmacogenetics: The Case of the Cytochrome P450 Isozymes

With the exception of lithium, the majority of psychotropics (as well as many nonpsychotropic drugs) are highly lipophilic; consequently, in order for these medications to be excreted from the body, they must undergo chemical transformation to make them less fat, and more water soluble. The metabolism and detoxification of the majority of modern chemotherapeutic agents, as well as a large number of foreign substances, is usually first achieved through oxidation by a group of isozymes belonging to the cytochrome P450 system. These structurally similar enzymes are widely distributed in the animal kingdom. The wide spread existence of these isozymes, as well as their similarities across species, testify to the vital importance of the cytochrome P450 system in the survival of organisms throughout the evolutionary ladder (Gonzalez, 1989, 1992; Kalow, 1993).

It is estimated that more than 20 P450 isozymes (grouped into families) exist in human beings, with each enzyme being encoded by a specific gene. Similar to the examples described above, the phenotypes (the activities of the enzymes) and genotypes (the structure of the encoding genes) of some of these P450 enzymes manifest distinct interindividual as well as cross-ethnic variations. Such diversity is most clearly seen in two extensively studied P450 isozymes, namely, the CYP2D6 (debrisoquin hydroxylase) and the CYP2C19 (mephenytoin hydroxylase). In any given population, these isozymes have been found to be bimodally distributed (as is also the case with other P450 enzymes). A certain proportion of people, deficient in the activity of these enzymes, are classified as poor metabolizers (PMs). In contrast, those without such deficiencies are classified as extensive metabolizers (EMs). It has been demonstrated that the bimodal distribution of the activities of these important enzymes is genetically controlled and can be traced to mutations in the nucleic acid sequence in the DNA, leading to alterations in the amino acid structure and subsequent activity of the enzymes.

Substantial cross-ethnic differences in the frequency of the PM phenotype exist with these enzymes (Kalow, 1992; Lin et al., 1993). Table 10.1 summarizes the frequency of PMs of both enzymes in studies involving different populations. The CYP2D6 PM rate ranges from less

TABLE 10.1. Ethnicity and Genetic Polymorphism of CYP2D6 and CYP2C19

	CYP2D6 (% PMs)	CYP2C19 (% PMs)
African Americans	1.9%	18.5%
African Blacks	0–8.1%	—
Amerindians	0–5.2%	0%
Asian Indians	—	20.8%
Caucasians	3–8.9%	2.5–6.7%
East Asians	0–2.4%	17.4–22%
Hispanics	1–4.5%	4.8%
Sans Bushman	19%	—

Note. Data from Lin and Poland (1995).

than 1% in some studies of Asians to as high as 19% among Sans Bushmen; limited data suggest that a relatively low frequency of PMs exist among Hispanics. Similarly, the CYP2C19 PM rate ranges from as low as 0% in Cuna Amerindians to 22% in Japanese. In addition, genotyping studies indicate that distinct patterns of mutations are responsible for the inactivation of the enzyme in PMs, as well as differential enzyme activities among EMs.

For example, although the rate of PMs for CYP2D6 was lower in Asians as compared to Caucasians, the majority of Asian EMs have significantly lower CYP2D6 enzyme activity as compared to Caucasian counterparts. A specific mutation (CYP2D6J) has recently been identified, which exists in up to 70% of Asians, but occurs rarely in Caucasians or African Blacks. Although this mutation does not completely inactivate the enzyme, it does render the enzyme less active. This effect is especially pronounced in approximately 30–40% of the Asians who are homozygotes for CYP2D6J (Wang, Huang, Lai, Liu, & Lai, 1993; Yakota et al., 1993). It should be noted that more than two dozen mutations of CYP2D6 have been identified, with multiple combinations of mutations observed. The resulting phenotypes are neither EMs or PMs but are somewhat intermediate. In addition, some subjects have multiple copies of CYP2D6 so that phenotypically, they are ultra-EMs or ultra-rapid metabolizers (Dahl, Johansson, Bertilsson, Ingelman-Sundberg, & Sjoqvist, 1995)

As shown in Table 10.2, with the exception of benzodiazepines (which are metabolized by other P450 isozymes) and lithium, CYP2D6 is involved in the metabolism of practically all medications commonly used in psychiatry, including most neuroleptics and antidepressants. Many studies have demonstrated that CYP2D6 activity correlates highly with the pharmacokinetics and clinical effects of its substrates

TABLE 10.2. Cytochrome P450 Isozymes and Their Most Common Substrates

CYP2D6	CYP2C19	CYP3A3/4	CYP1A2
Amitriptyline	Amitriptyline	Amitriptyline	Amitriptyline
Imipramine	Imipramine	Imipramine	Imipramine
Clomipramine	Clomipramine	Clomipramine	Clomipramine
Desipramine	Diazepam	Alprazolam	Caffeine
Maprotiline	Hexobarbital	Triazolam	Clozapine
Nortriptyline	Moclobemide	Midazolam	Tacrine
Fluoxetine		Nefazodone	Haloperidol
Paroxetine		Sertraline	Fluvoxamine
Trazodone		Carbamazepine	
Venlafaxine			
Haloperidol			
Perphenazine			
Risperidone			
Thioridazine			
Propranolol	Propranolol	Terfenadine	Theophylline
Codeine	Mephenytoin	Astemizole	Phenacetin
Dextromethorphan	Warfarin	Cisapride	Verapamil
	Tolbutamide	Verapamil	
		Nifedipine	
		Erythromycin	
		Lidocaine	
		Quinidine	

Note. Data from Nemeroff et al. (1996) and Riesenman (1995).

(Llerena, Alm, Dahl, Ekqvist, & Bertilsson, 1992; Pollock, 1994). CYP2D6 PMs consistently exhibit significantly higher concentrations of neuroleptics and tricyclic antidepressants (TCAs) when treated with similar doses of the medications. Among CYP2D6 EMs, a strong negative correlation often exists between the enzyme activity and the concentration of the substrates. For example, in a study involving the administration of test doses of haloperidol, PMs experienced severe extrapyramidal side effects and had significantly higher serum haloperidol concentrations (Llerena et al., 1992).

As seen in Table 10.2, CYP2C19 metabolizes different medications than does CYP2D6. In reality, both enzymes may share in the metabolism of the same medication (e.g., many TCAs), with one isozyme being the primary metabolic route. The polymorphic nature of this enzyme has been known for over a decade, and recently two specific mutations responsible for the PM status were identified. As seen in Table 10.1, there is a different pattern of the frequency of PMs with CYP2C19 compared to CYP2D6. As shown in Table 10.1, PMs are quite frequent among Asians and African Americans but less frequent in Caucasians. As shown in Table 10.2, CYP2C19 is involved in the metabolism of the anxiolytic, diazepam. A higher rate of PMs of this enzyme in Asians thus should lead to slower metabolism of diazepam in a significant number of patients in this ethnic group, and a number of clinical reports have indicated that Asians tended to tolerate significantly lower doses of diazepam and often reported a higher rate of sedating side effects.

In contrast to the two enzymes discussed above, there is no clear evidence of polymorphism with regard to CYP3A4 and CYP1A2, two other cytochrome P450 isozymes that also are important for the metabolism of psychotropics, particularly those used to treat anxiety disorders, for example, several benzodiazepines, TCAs, and selective serotonin reuptake inhibitors (SSRIs) (DeVane, 1994; Kalow, 1992). However, some evidence of ethnic differences in the activity of these enzymes does exist. For example, the calcium channel blocker nifedipine, a substrate for CYP3A4, is reported to be metabolized more slowly in South and East Asians and Hispanics (Ahsan et al., 1993; Castaneda-Hernandez, Hoyo-Vadillo, Palma-Aguirre, & Flores-Murrieta, 1993).

Because the activity of CYP1A2 can be increased by constituents of tobacco, charcoal-broiled beef, cruciferous vegetables, and industrial toxins, and CYP3A4 activity can be both increased (e.g., by steroids, carbamazepine) as well as competitively inhibited by a number of agents (e.g., naringin, an ingredient of grapefruit juice), differences among ethnic groups in the expression of these enzymes are commonly believed to be environmentally rather than genetically determined. This has been demonstrated in a number of pharmacokinetic studies of theophylline and antipyrine in Sudanese and Asian Indians. While residing in their home country and eating a vegetarian diet, they manifested a significantly slower metabolic rate of these substances. However, when they moved to London, and presumably changed their diet to include meat, their pharmacokinetic profiles became indistinguishable from those for the British whites (Branch, Salih, & Homeida, 1978). A study comparing the pharmacokinetics of clomipramine between Asian Indians and British whites also showed similar ethnic contrasts that could be explained at least in part by differences in dietary habits (Allen, Rack, & Vaddadi, 1977).

Ethnicity and Other Pharmacokinetic Factors

A number of other pharmacokinetic factors also have been demonstrated to contribute to ethnic differences in the biotransformation of drugs, though none have been studied as extensively as the cytochrome system. Recent studies (Kalow, 1992) indicate that cytochrome P450 isozymes also exist in the central nervous system (CNS), and it is conceivable that ethnic variations in P450 isozymes also may exist at the CNS level, leading to differential drug responses not readily explained by peripheral pharmacokinetics. Protein binding represents another important factor in the distribution of many drugs, as variations in the concentration of these drug-binding proteins in plasma can significantly influence the effect of the drug by changing the concentration of the free (unbound) fraction (Levy & Moreland, 1984). Because usually only the free fraction of the drug is pharmacologically active and capable of crossing the blood–brain barrier, changes in the concentrations of drug-binding proteins might have clinical significance (Crabtree, Jann, & Pitts, 1991). The structures of these plasma proteins are genetically determined, exhibit polymorphism, and have been shown to vary across ethnic groups in several studies (Juneja, Weitkamp, Stratil, Gahne, & Guttormsen, 1988). However, cross-ethnic studies (Crabtree et al., 1991) of plasma protein-binding have revealed conflicting results, and thus the contribution that plasma protein-binding has to different responses across ethnic groups remains to be determined. Finally, the fat content of the body, which may differ across ethnic groups, can lead to differences in the volume of distribution and thus the pharmacokinetics of drugs that are lipophilic. This, in fact, has been identified as one of the reasons for the greater effect of diazepam in Asians as compared to Caucasians (Kumana, Ler, Chan, Ko, & Lin, 1987).

Ethnicity and Pharmacodynamics

Although much less understood and discussed, substantial interindividual and cross-ethnic differences in pharmacodynamics also exist. One of the classical examples is the mydriatic (pupillary enlargement) responses to various classes of drugs including cocaine, ephedrine, atropine and scopolamine (Angenent & Koelle, 1953; Garde, Aston, Endler, & Sison, 1978). Blacks have been shown to be consistently least responsive to these local mydriatics, followed by Asians, with Caucasians falling on the other extreme. This reduction in the mydriatic effect correlated with the degree of pigmentation of the iris, and was not seen among albino Africans. Beta-blockers, such as propranolol, have been found to be relatively ineffective in treating hypertension in African American patients (Moser & Lunn, 1981), and the doses of propranolol required for the effective treatment of hypertension in Asians were substantially smaller than in Caucasians (Zhou, Koshakji, Siolberstein, Wilkinson, & Wood, 1989). Recent studies objectively demonstrated that the effects of propranolol on blood pressure and heart rate were most pronounced in Asians, and least prominent in African Americans, with Caucasians falling in between (Dimsdale, Ziegler, & Graham, 1988), differences that could not be explained by pharmacokinetic factors (Zhou et al., 1989). Studies demonstrating that blacks have significantly higher concentrations of cyclic AMP, both at baseline and after the administration of propranolol, suggest that blacks might have a higher degree of beta-adrenoceptor activity (Rutledge, Steinberg, & Cardozo, 1989). This in turn has led to the hypothesis that differences in the sensitivity of adrenoceptors might be the major cause for the differential effects of propranolol and other beta-blockers in various ethnic groups (Kalow, 1989). The degree to which this might affect the use of beta-blocking agents in such disorders as social phobia, or as an adjunct in treating panic disorder, is not known.

ETHNICITY AND PSYCHOTROPIC RESPONSE

Since the 1950s, there have been frequent reports of ethnic differences in psychotropic response, which until recently have been mostly based on clinical impressions and surveys (Lin et al., 1993). However, in the last decade increasing numbers of researchers have started to utilize more vigorous study designs to link these clinical reports with the pharmacokinetic and pharmacodynamic mechanisms discussed above. Some of the more representative studies of this nature will be highlighted below.

Neuroleptics

Perhaps the most extensive work has been done with antipsychotic medications. Because these drugs have only a limited role in the treatment of anxiety disorders, this literature will briefly be discussed here. The pharmacokinetics and pharmacodynamics of haloperidol have been demonstrated to differ significantly between Asians and Caucasians. When given comparable doses of medication, Asian schizophrenic patients (Potkin et al., 1984) and normal volunteers (Lin, Poland, Lau, & Rubin, 1988) exhibited plasma haloperidol concentrations that were approximately 50% greater than their Caucasian counterparts. Midha, Hawes, Hubbard, Korchinski, and McKay (1988a, 1988b) found no difference between Canadian blacks and whites in the pharmacokinetics of two phenothiazines, while Jann, Lam, and Chang (1993) reported significantly different pharmacokinetic profiles of haloperidol for Chinese and African Americans as compared to Caucasians and Hispanics.

The mechanisms responsible for such ethnic differences are currently an active area of research. Because the phenotype and genotype of CYP2D6 differ significantly across ethnic groups, it has been suggested that this isozyme may contribute to ethnic differences in the pharmacokinetics of haloperidol. Other studies investigating the metabolic pathway of haloperidol suggest additional reasons for these ethnic differences (Chang, Chen, Lee, Hu, & Yeh, 1987; Jann et al., 1993). In the above-mentioned study with normal volunteers (Lin, Poland, et al., 1988), as well as a study with Asian schizophrenic patients (Lin et al., 1989), results suggested that pharmacodynamic differences also may exist.

Tricyclic Antidepressants

In contrast to neuroleptics, studies of ethnic differences in the pharmacokinetics of the TCAs have led to inconclusive results (Silver, Poland, & Lin, 1993). Among previous studies comparing Asians with Caucasians, some revealed that Asians metabolize TCAs significantly more slowly than their Caucasian counterparts (Kishimoto & Hollister, 1984; Rudorfer, Lane, Chang, Zhang, & Potter, 1984). However, other studies showed differences in the same direction, but these did not reach statistical significance, particularly after controlling for body weight (Pi, Simpson, & Cooper, 1986; Pi et al., 1989). In a recently completed study, Lin et al. (1997) compared the pharmacokinetics of imipramine among Asians, African Americans, Hispanics, and Caucasians. With the exception of higher desipramine concentrations in the African American group, they did not find any significant differences among the four comparison groups. These results are in congruence with an earlier study demonstrating lack of difference in the pharmacokinetics of nortriptyline between Mexican Americans and Caucasians (Gaviria, Gil, & Javaid, 1986). The elevation of secondary amine concentrations also has been previously reported among African American patients (Ziegler & Biggs, 1977).

Pharmacodynamic factors have not been formally examined in studies comparing the use of antidepressants across ethnic groups. However, results from two clinical studies in Asia (Hu, Lee, Yang, & Tseng, 1983; Yamashita & Asano, 1979) indicate that severely depressed, hospitalized Asian patients respond clinically to lower combined concentrations of imipramine and desipramine (130 ng/ml) than previously reported in North American and European studies (180–200 ng/ml), thereby suggesting that differential brain receptor responsivity might also play a role in determining ethnic differences in TCA dosage requirements. Our own work has shown that Asians, and to a lesser extent Hispanics, appear to be more sensitive to the stimulatory effects of TCAs (an unwanted side effect) and to display increased prolactin and cortisol levels as well. Although clinical reports suggest that African Americans are more susceptible to CNS side effects of TCAs (Livingston, Zucker, Isenberg, & Wetzel, 1983; Rudorfer & Robins, 1982), the mechanisms that might be responsible for such a phenomenon have not been carefully evaluated.

Despite the fact that SSRIs and other newer classes of antidepressants are recognized as being metabolized through the cytochrome P450 system, there have not been cross-cultural studies with these medications.

Benzodiazepines and Other Anxiolytics

Confirming earlier clinical and survey reports, controlled studies involving Asians and Caucasians demonstrated significant pharmacokinetic differences between the two ethnic groups (Ghoneim et al., 1981; Kumana et al., 1987; Lin, Lau, Smith, & Poland, 1988; Zhang, Reviriego, Lou, Sjoqvist, & Bertilsson, 1990). Three of the studies, conducted in Asians residing in different areas of the world, used diazepam as the test drug, while one utilized alprazolam. Given the diversity of sites and research methodology, the consistency in these reports of a slower metabolism of benzodiazepines suggests that genetic factors are more important than environmental factors in the control of benzodiazepine metabolism.

In a recent study of the pharmacokinetics and pharmacodynamics of adinazolam, a triazolo-benzodiazepine currently being investigated as an anxiolytic and antidepressant, African Americans were found to have both increased clearance of adinazolam, resulting in significantly higher concentrations of N-desmethyladinazolam, a metabolite of adinazolam, and greater drug effects on psychomotor performance (Fleishaker, Smith, Friedman, & Hulst, 1992; Lin et al., 1993). N-desmethyladinazolam has been shown primarily to mediate the benzodiazepine-like side effects, including effects on psychomotor performance, after adinazolam administration. This might explain the greater drug effects observed in some African Americans. However, a more recent study by our group (Ajir et al., 1997). showed that Asians had the highest plasma levels of adinazolam and its metabolite, with no differences in pharmacodynamic responses. Future studies with larger number of subjects are necessary to sort out these discrepancies.

To our knowledge, there are no published data regarding the cytochrome system and buspirone, a nonbenzodiazepine antianxiety agent.

Lithium

Again, though lithium is not a treatment of choice for anxiety disorders, we will briefly review the work on ethnic differences for this medication. Several cross-national comparison studies have established the use of lower doses of lithium as well as lower therapeutic lithium levels among Asians (Lin et al., 1993). Thus, it appears that, compared to their Caucasian counterparts, Asian bipolar patients may require lower doses of lithium because of pharmacodynamic reasons, or more specifically, increased CNS responsivity.

The distribution of lithium across cellular membranes is controlled by several membrane transport and countertransport mechanisms, and the sodium-lithium countertransport system appears to play a particularly important role. This system is significantly less active among African Americans and African blacks as compared to Caucasians; this might contribute to a higher red blood cell (RBC)/serum lithium ratio among blacks (Okpaku, Frazer, & Mendels, 1980; Strickland, Lin, Fu, Anderson, & Zheng, 1995). Because the intracellular concentration of lithium may determine its clinical and side effects, ethnic differences in the RBC/serum lithium ratio may have important clinical significance.

CULTURE AND "NONBIOLOGICAL" ISSUES

In contrast to the technological progress made in the biological arena, less progress has been made in regard to the cultural and nonbiological issues surrounding the giving and taking of medications. Consequently, our understanding of these extremely important issues remains fragmented and is not scientifically based. The prescription and taking of medication is primarily a social process. Thus, the effect of medication is deeply influenced by the symbolic nature of the transactions and interactions between physicians and patients, as well as by those important in their social networks. Irrespective of the category of medication, treatment outcome often is determined only to some extent by the "true" pharmacological properties of the chemical substances used, and also to a degree by the result of the interplay among various cultural influences. In the following, some of the most salient issues will be discussed briefly.

Assessment of psychiatric patients in cross-cultural settings often results in misdiagnosis and inappropriate treatment decisions. This was most clearly demonstrated in a series of studies that consistently demonstrated that African American patients were more likely to be assigned a more severe diagnosis such as schizophrenia, to be treated with neuroleptics irrespective of diagnosis, and to be given significantly higher doses of neuroleptics compared to other ethnic groups (D'Mello, McNeil, & Harris, 1989; Price, Glazer, & Morgenstern, 1985; Zito, Craig, Wanderling, & Seigel, 1987). They also were significantly more likely to be placed on depot rather than oral medications, presumably reflecting the clinicians' heightened concern with problems of compliance. This tendency to "overdiagnose" and "overtreat" African Americans is likely one of the reasons for the higher prevalence of tardive dyskinesia often observed among African American psychiatric patients. Another example pertains to the influence of language on diagnosis. When a group of Spanish-speaking patients in a state hospital were reinterviewed by language- and cultural-congruent clinicians, using standardized criteria for diagnoses, a substantial number of diagnoses were changed from schizophrenia to psychotic depression. This resulted in a change in medications and a much better outcome for these patients (Lawson, Herrera, & Costa, 1992).

The Influence of Stress and Social Support on Drug Responses

Culture strongly influences the type and level of stress, as well as the structure and function of social networks (Comas-Díaz & Griffith, 1988; Kirmayer & Robbins, 1991; Lin, 1987), with stress and social support serving as important mediating factors affecting the prognosis and outcome of treatment. People with a higher level of stress and lower degree of social support are more likely to become mentally ill (Lidwig & Collete, 1970; Myers, Lindenthal, Pepper, & Ostrander, 1972), less likely to be compliant with prescribed medication (Nelson, Stason, Neutra, & Solomon, 1980), and more likely to have poorer clinical outcome (Jablensky et al., 1992; Lin & Kleinman, 1988). In addition, alterations in the level of stress and the availability of social support also may change the therapeutic dosages and therapeutic concentration ranges of different psychotropics, as was shown by Lieberman and Strauss (1984) with bipolar patients who needed higher doses of lithium to maintain remission when under extreme social stress.

Another factor that may have importance here is the concept of "expressed emotion" (EE), characterized by frequent criticism, hostility, and emotional overinvolvement, which has been studied cross culturally on a limited basis. For example, it has been reported that Hispanic families tend to have significantly lower EE ratings as compared to Anglo Americans and the British (Jenkins & Karno, 1992; Keefe, Padilla, & Carlos, 1978). Several well-designed studies examining the effect of

EE have found that patients with high EE family members were significantly more likely to relapse (Anderson, Reiss, & Hogarty, 1986; Falloon, Boyd, & McGill, 1984) and to be subsequently treated with higher doses of the same medication (Falloon & Liberman, 1983; Hogarty et al., 1988). It is possible that such cultural differences in family atmosphere may have important influences on drug responsiveness across cultures.

Compliance Issues

Noncompliance is a major problem in the treatment of chronic medical conditions and psychiatric disorders as well. Several recent studies have found that compliance to psychotropics may be more problematic among non-Western populations (Smith, Lin, & Mendoza, 1993). One major reason for this could be the divergence in beliefs and the communication difficulties between patients and clinicians who are not of the same background. The results of a study in South Africa provide a dramatic example (Gillis, Trollip, Jakoet, & Holden, 1987). In this study, 406 patients belonging to three ethnic groups (white, black, and "colored") were followed for a 2-year period after discharge from a psychiatric hospital. The results showed that approximately two thirds of black patients, one half of colored patients, and one quarter of white patients were noncompliant for oral phenothiazines. The authors noted that understanding of the treatment protocols by the relatives of the black and colored families was particularly poor. The results can be explained by multiple interacting variables including discrimination, the possibility of culture and communication mismatch, and the impact of structural barriers such as cost and availability of transportation. Perhaps for analogous reasons, African Americans are reportedly less compliant (D'Mello et al., 1989) and consequently more likely to be placed on injectable antipsychotics (Price et al., 1985).

A study of an Asian refugee population performed by Kinzie, Leung, Boehnlein, and Fleck (1987) serves to illustrate further the problems with medication compliance in ethnic populations. They found that, despite being given adequate supplies of TCAs, 61% of their depressed patients showed no detectable plasma levels and another 24% revealed only very low TCA plasma levels. When questioned, these patients admitted to being noncompliant for a variety of reasons. After a program of education regarding the importance of long-term medication and the maintenance of appropriate blood levels, there was a significant improvement in compliance in some, but not all, refugee groups.

Placebo Effects

The placebo effect is commonly regarded as being responsible for 30–70% of the therapeutic responses observed in clinical settings, including trials for panic disorder and generalized anxiety disorder. Unfortunately, the results of large-scale clinical trials do not discuss whether there is a differential placebo response across ethnicity. Our limited experience indicates that this might be true. In a small study of patients having panic disorder with agoraphobia using a novel anxiolytic medication, subjects were given placebo for 2 weeks prior to active medication. Those whose symptoms improved below entrance criteria during this time were not entered into the study. There were 3 of 10 Hispanic patients and 1 of 20 Caucasian patients considered placebo responders, suggesting a differential placebo response; this deserves further study in large-scale clinical trials.

Other than its inclusion in controlled drug trials, the placebo effect has received minimal attention both in medical practice and in research (Kleinman, 1988; White, Tursky, & Schwartz, 1985). Yet such factors as color, size, preparation, and method of drug administration (Buckalew & Coffield, 1982; Jacobs & Nordan, 1979; Rabkin et al., 1990) may significantly influence the extent of placebo responses. A few examples highlight how placebo response may differ according to culture and ethnicity. Escobar and Tuason (1980) conducted a cross-national study on the efficacy of trazodone and imipramine compared to placebo in Colombian and North American depressed patients. They found that Colombian patients improved more than those in the United States both with the antidepressants and placebo. Interestingly, color of the capsules appears to exert differential placebo effects in different ethnic groups. Buckalew and Coffield (1982) reported that white capsules were seen by white subjects as analgesics, yet blacks viewed them as stimulants. In contrast, black capsules were regarded as stimulants by whites and as analgesics by blacks. An extension of the placebo effect can be seen in reports showing an increased number of unwanted side effects in non-Caucasians, over and above what could be explained by more traditional biological factors (Escobar & Tuason, 1980; Lin & Shen, 1991; Marcus & Cancro, 1982).

Simultaneous Use of Traditional and/or Alternative Healing Methods

Throughout the world, as well as across all ethnic groups in the United States, traditional herbal medicines continue to be extensively utilized, often side by side with modern Western pharmaceutical agents (Chan & Chang, 1976; Kleinman, 1980; Westermeyer, 1989a, 1989b). Contrary to the beliefs of most physicians, many of these herbal drugs are pharmacologically active, capable of producing significant interactions with prescribed drugs (Shader & Greenblatt, 1988). As examples (see Smith et al., 1993), the anticholinergic properties inherent in the Japanese herbs *Swertia japonica* and *kamikihi-to* and the Cuban folk medicine *Datura candida* may cause atropine psychosis, particularly when ingested concomitantly with TCAs or low-potency neuroleptics. Because of its high concentration of caffeine, the South American holly, *Ilex guayusa*, can counteract the sedative and anxiolytic effects of benzodiazepines and related compounds. Concurrent use of the Nigerian root extract of *Schumanniophyton problematicum*, a popular treatment for psychosis among Nigerians, with sedative hypnotics or neuroleptics may lead to potentiation of tranquilizing effects. Several Chinese herbs, including the popular ginseng, have been found to have potent effects (both stimulating and inhibiting) on the cytochrome P450 enzymes (Liu, 1991). Increased awareness on the part of clinicians and further clarification of the biological effects remain important as patients continue to rely on these traditional herbs as an adjunct to pharmacotherapy. The following case report highlights some of these issues.

Ms. A. was a 28-year-old Hispanic female of Mexican descent who presented with a 6-week history of depressive symptoms. She was placed on an SSRI with minimal side effects and a good response. After 8 weeks of treatment, Ms. A. called, stating that she no longer wanted to take the SSRI because she believed that it had caused anxiety, irritability, and insomnia. Further inquiry revealed that Ms. A was frustrated with the progress of the treatment and, following the advice of a cousin, had started to take a combination of traditional herbal medicines in addition to her antidepressant. This combination consisted of pills and teas of two herbs, valerian and tilla. She took these herbs for a week before stopping abruptly due to the excessive sedation. Within a day of stopping she was overwhelmed with the anxiety symptoms that had precipitated her call. She attributed these symptoms to the SSRI she was taking.

The symptoms she described were unlikely to have been caused by an SSRI that had been well tolerated for 8 weeks. A much more likely explanation was the abrupt discontinuation of the herbal medicine. Tilla is a compound with benzodiazepine-like action and valerian has activity at the gamma-aminobutyric acid receptor on which benzodiazepines act. Her sedation was probably due to the combination of these drugs, whereas her anxiety symptoms were a result of her abrupt discontinuation and constituted a withdrawal syndrome.

The patient was reassured that the symptoms were not due to the SSRI, but rather to her stopping the herbal medication. She was restarted on the SSRI and provided with medication for sleep. After a few days the anxiety symptoms had resolved.

This case points out two important factors that can affect response to pharmacological agents: misattribution of side effects and concomitant use of herbal medication. Herbal medication often is viewed as milder than "Western" medications and its interactions with more traditional medications may not be understood. Although the patient had tolerated 8 weeks of treatment without incident, and developed the withdrawal symptoms after stopping the herbal drugs, she attributed the side effects to the SSRI.

CLINICAL GUIDELINES

Despite the progress described in this chapter, formal study of the field of ethnicity and pharmacology is, if not in its infancy, then still in early childhood. Because of this, it is difficult to formulate guidelines that should be followed by clinicians treating patients of different ethnicities. In addition, the published work often pertains to medications that were the standard of care at the time (e.g., TCAs) but may have been supplanted by newer medications (e.g., SSRIs). In fact, there are no controlled studies of the newer antidepressants where the influence of ethnicity on drug response has been assessed. This is unfortunate, as these newer medications have become treatments of choice for depression, as well as for many of the anxiety disorders.

Good clinical practice dictates listening to the patient. If a patient is experiencing untoward side effects at a dose that one might think is "too low" to produce those side effects, consider that the person may be a PM and have a higher plasma level than would have been predicted. These patients may cluster within certain ethnic groups, particularly Asians, and perhaps for benzodiazepines, African Americans. However, because of the tremendous overlap among subjects in each ethnic group, no strict guidelines regarding dosing can be provided. Although it is important to consider ethnicity as a factor in drug dosing and side effects, this should not be adhered to in a rigid fashion. One danger in blindly accepting the reports discussed above is that significant cross-ethnic/cross-cultural differences in psychotropic drug responses could be interpreted stereotypically, leading to a scenario where all patients from an ethnic group are always treated with, for example, lower doses. This would not take into account the large interindividual variation, even within an specific ethnic group.

Although it has not been studied systematically, another area that may differentially affect patients from ethnic groups is that of drug interactions. Because many different medications (psychotropic and others) are metabolized by the same P450 isozymes, there may be competition for the enzyme's activity. If a patient is a slow metabolizer (SM) or even an EM of one drug (e.g., a TCA) and he or she is given another drug metabolized through the same system (e.g., an SSRI), the blood levels of the TCA may be markedly elevated because its metabolism is slowed secondary to the competition with the metabolism of the SSRI. Many drug interactions are now understood to be partially a function of this process. For example, if multiple medications metabolized by CYP2D6 are used concomitantly in a SM or EM, they may develop toxic plasma levels of one or the other agent. It is important to recognize that nonpsychotropic medications also are metabolized by these same isozymes (see the lower part of Table 10.2), and care must be taken to find out all medications a patient is taking. This is particularly important in elderly patients, who not only take multiple medications but in whom the metabolic processes are slowed down. Drug interactions in this group are very problematic, leading to multiple behavioral syndromes, and could even be life threatening.

In addition to these considerations, it is important to elicit the patient's expectations and beliefs about what the medication will do, both in positive and negative directions. Finally, it should be noted that families can play a major role in the process of taking medication. Asian, Hispanic, and African American families may have unique approaches to illness behavior and taking medication, and these may be at variance with what is considered "traditional" Caucasian family behavior.

SUMMARY AND CONCLUSIONS

The literature reviewed above clearly indicates that ethnicity and culture are important variables that significantly influence the effect of psychotropics. Mechanisms responsible for such differences include not only those belonging to the realm of pharmacokinetics and pharmacodynamics, but also various psychosocial factors. Despite remarkable recent progress, much remains unclarified, and research in this area will continue to be of great importance.

Ethnic and cultural considerations have assumed increasing relevance in the process of drug development. Traditionally, the safety and efficacy of pharmaceutical agents are usually tested only in selected groups, most often younger, Caucasian males, but the results are extrapolated to other populations. As shown in many examples above, this would appear to be insufficient. Efforts need to be made to recruit more subjects from multiple ethnic groups into drug trials, although this may be hampered by the reluctance of members from minority groups to participate in research (Neal & Turner, 1991).

Finally, ethnic differences and similarities in response to psychoactive agents provide a dramatic example of how cultural and biological diversities often interact with each other, and how these diversities might serve as a stimulus for new discoveries. This is easily seen by the development of the field of pharmacogenetics. It is to be expected that interest in these issues will continue, with cross-ethnic research designs serving as a powerful tool for psychopharmacological research in the future.

ACKNOWLEDGMENTS

This work was supported by the National Institute of Mental Health Research Center on the Psychobiology of Ethnicity (Grant Nos. MH 47193 and MH 34471), National Institute of Mental Health Research Scientist Development Award No. MH 00534 to Russell E. Poland and National Institutes of Health General Clinical Research Center Grant No. RR00425.

REFERENCES

Ahsan, C. H., Renwick, A. G., Waller, D. G., Challenor, V. F., George, C. F., & Amanullah, M. (1993). The influence of dose and ethnic origins on the pharmacokinetics of nifedipine. *Clinical Pharmacology and Therapeutics, 54*, 329–328.

Ajir, K., Smith, M., Lin, K. M., Poland, R. E., Fleishaker, J. C., Chambers, J. H., Anderson, D., Nuccio, C., Zheng, Y. P. (1997). The pharamacokinetics and pharmacodynamics of adinazolam: Multi-ethnic comparisons. *Psychopharmacology, 129*, 265–270.

Allen, J. J., Rack, P. H., & Vaddadi, K. S. (1977). Differences in the effects of clomipramine on English and Asian volunteers: Preliminary report on a pilot study. *Postgraduate Medicine, 53*, 79–86.

Anderson, C. M., Reiss, D. J., & Hogarty, G. E. (1986). *Schizophrenia and the family: A practitioner's guide to psychoeducation and management.* New York: Guilford Press.

Angenent, W. J., & Koelle, G. B. (1953). A possible enzymatic basis for the differential action of mydriatics on light and dark irises. *Journal of Physiology, 119*, 102–117.

Argawal, D. P., & Goedde, H. W. (1990). *Alcohol metabolism, alcohol intolerance and alcoholism.* Berlin: Springer-Verlag.

Branch, R. A., Salih, S. Y., & Homeida, M. (1978). Racial differences in drug metabolizing ability: A study with antipyrine in the Sudan. *Clinical Pharmacology and Therapeutics, 24,* 283–286.

Buckalew, L. W., & Coffield, K. E. (1982). Drug expectations associated with perceptual characteristics: Ethnic factors. *Perceptual and Motor Skills, 55,* 915–918.

Castaneda-Hernandez, G., Hoyo-Vadillo, C., Palma-Aguirre, J. A., & Flores-Murrieta, F. J. (1993). Pharmacokinetics of oral nifedipine in different populations. *Journal of Clinical Pharmacology, 33,* 140–145.

Chan, C. W., & Chang, J. K. (1976). The role of Chinese medicine in New York City's Chinatown. *American Journal of Chinese Medicine, 4,* 31–45, 129–146.

Chang, W.-H., Chen, T.-Y., Lee, C.-F., Hu, W. H., & Yeh, E. K. (1987). Low plasma reduced haloperidol/haloperidol ratios in Chinese patients. *Biological Psychiatry, 22,* 1406–1408.

Comas-Diáz, L., & Griffith, E. E. H. (Eds.). (1988). *Clinical guidelines in cross-cultural mental health.* New York: Wiley.

Crabtree, B. L., Jann, M. W., & Pitts, W. M. (1991). Alpha₁ acid glycoprotein levels in patients with schizophrenia: Effect of treatment with haloperidol. *Biological Psychiatry, 29,* 43A–185A.

Dahl, M. L., Johansson, I., Bertilsson, L., Ingelman-Sundberg, M., & Sjoqvist, F. (1995). Ultra-rapid hydroxylation of debrisoquine in a Swedish population: Analysis of the molecular genetic basis. *Journal of Pharmacology and Experimental Therapeutics, 274,* 516–520.

DeVane, C. L. (1994). Pharmacokinetics of the newer antidepressants: Clinical relevance. *American Journal of Medicine, 97*(6A), 13S–23S.

Dimsdale, J., Ziegler, M., & Graham, R. (1988). The effect of hypertension, sodium, and race on isoproterenol sensitivity. *Clinical and Experimental Hypertension—Theory and Practice, A10,* 747–756.

D'Mello, D. A., McNeil, J. A., & Harris, W. (1989, May). *Multiethnic variance in psychiatric diagnosis and neuroleptic dosage.* Paper presented at the 142th annual meeting of the American Psychiatric Association in San Francisco, CA.

Escobar, J. I., & Tuason, V. B. (1980). Antidepressant agents: A cross cultural study. *Psychopharmacology Bulletin, 16,* 49–52.

Falloon, I. R. H., Boyd, J. L., & McGill, C. W. (Eds.). (1984). *Family care of schizophrenia: A problem-solving approach to the treatment of mental illness.* New York: Guilford Press.

Falloon, I. R. H., & Liberman, R. P. (1983). Interactions between drug and psychosocial therapy in schizophrenia. *Schizophrenia Bulletin, 9,* 543–554.

Fleishaker, J. C., Smith, T. C., Friedman, H. L., & Hulst, L. K. (1992). Separation of the pharmacokinetic/pharmacodynamic properties of oral and IV adinazolam mesylate and N-desmethyladinazolam mesylate in healthy volunteers. *Drug Investigations, 4,* 155–165.

Garde, J. F., Aston, R., Endler, G. C., & Sison, O. S. (1978). Racial mydriatic response to belladonna premedication. *Anesthesia and Analgesia, 57,* 572–576.

Gaviria, M., Gil, A. A., & Javaid, J. I. (1986). Nortriptyline kinetics in Hispanic and Anglo subjects. *Journal of Clinical Psychopharmacology, 6,* 227–231.

Ghoneim, M. M., Korttila, K., Chiang, C. K., Jacobs, L., Schoenwald, R. D., Newaldt, S. P., & Lauaba, K. O. (1981). Diazepam effects and kinetics in Caucasians and Orientals. *Clinical Pharmacology and Therapeutics, 29,* 749–756.

Gillis, L. S., Trollip, D., Jakoet, A., & Holden, T. (1987). Non-compliance with psychotropic medication. *South African Medical Journal, 72,* 602–606.

Gonzalez, F. J. (1989). The molecular biology of cytochrome P450s. *Pharmacological Reviews, 40,* 243–288.

Gonzalez, F. J. (1992). Human cytochromes P450: Problems and prospects. *TiPS Reviews, 13,* 346–352.

Greenblatt, D. J. (1993). Basic pharmacokinetic principles and their application to psychotropic drugs. *Journal of Clinical Psychiatry, 54*(Suppl.), 8–13.

Hogarty, G. E., McEvoy, J. P., Munetz, M., DiBarry, A. L., Bartone, P., Cather, R., Cooley, S. J., Ulrich, R. F., Carter, M., & Madonia, M. J. (1988). Dose of fluphenazine, familial expressed emotion, and outcome in schizophrenia. *Archives of General Psychiatry, 45,* 797–805.

Hu, W. H., Lee, C. F., Yang, Y. Y., & Tseng, Y. T. (1983). Imipramine plasma levels and clinical response. *Bulletin of the Chinese Society of Neurology and Psychiatry, 9,* 40–49.

Jablensky, A., Sartorius, N., Ernberg, G., Anker, M., Korten, A., Cooper, J. E., Day, R., & Bertelsen, A. (1992). Schizophrenia: Manifestations, incidence and course in different cultures: A World Health Organization ten-country study. *Psychological Medicine, 20,* 1–97.

Jacobs, K. W., & Nordan, F. M. (1979). Classification of placebo drugs: Effect of color. *Perceptual and Motor Skills, 49,* 367–372.

Jann, M. W., Lam, Y. W., & Chang, W. H. (1993). Haloperidol and reduced haloperidol plasma concentrations in different ethnic populations and interindividual variabilities in haloperidol metabolism. In K. M. Lin, R. E. Poland, & G. Nakasaki (Eds.), *Psychopharmacology and psychobiology of ethnicity* (pp. 133–152). Washington, DC: American Psychiatric Press.

Jenkins, J. H., & Karno, M. (1992). The meaning of expressed emotion: Theoretical issues raised by cross-cultural research. *American Journal of Psychiatry, 149,* 9–21.

Juneja, R. K., Weitkamp, L. R., Stratil, A., Gahne, B., & Guttormsen, S. A. (1988). Further studies of the plasma α B-glycoprotein polymorphism: Two new alleles and allele frequencies in Caucasians and in American Blacks. *Human Heredity, 38,* 267–272.

Kalow, W. (1989). Race and therapeutic drug response. *New England Journal of Medicine, 320,* 588–589.

Kalow, W. (1990). Pharmacogenetics: Past and future. *Life Sciences, 47,* 1385–1397.

Kalow, W. (1991). Interethnic variation of drug metabolism. *Trends in Pharmacological Sciences, 12,* 102–107.

Kalow, W. (Ed.). (1992). *Pharmacogenetics of drug metabolism.* New York: Pergamon Press.

Kalow, W. (1993). Pharmacogenetics: Its biologic roots and the medical challenge. *Clinical Pharmacology and Therapeutics, 54,* 235–241.

Keefe, S. E., Padilla, A. M., & Carlos, M. L. (1978). *Emotional support systems in two cultures: A comparison of Mexican-Americans and Anglo Americans.* (Available from University of California-Los Angeles, Spanish Speaking Mental Health Center)

Kinzie, J. D., Leung, P., Boehnlein, J., & Fleck, J. (1987). Tricyclic antidepressant plasma levels in Indochinese refugees: Clinical implication. *Journal of Nervous and Mental Disorders, 175,* 480–485.

Kirmayer, L. J., & Robbins, J. M. (1991). *Current concepts of somatization, research and clinical perspectives.* Washington, DC: American Psychiatric Press.

Kishimoto, A., & Hollister, L. E. (1984). Nortriptyline kinetics in Japanese and Americans [Letter to the editor]. *Journal of Clinical Psychopharmacology, 4,* 171–172.

Kleinman, A. (1980). *Patients and healers in the context of culture.* Berkeley: University of California Press.

Kleinman, A. (1988). *Rethinking psychiatry.* New York: Free Press.

Kumana, C. R., Ler, I. J., Chan, M., Ko, W., & Lin, H. J. (1987). Differences in diazepam pharmacokinetics in Chinese and White Caucasians—Relation to body lipid stores. *European Journal of Clinical Pharmacology, 32,* 211–215.

Lawson, W. B., Herrera, J. M., & Costa, J. (1992). The dexamethasone suppression test as an adjunct in diagnosing depression. *Journal of the Association for Academic Minority Physicians, 3,* 17–19.

Lesser, I. M., Lin, K. M., & Poland, R. E. (1994). Ethnic differences in the response to psychotropic drugs. In S. Friedman (Ed.), *Anxiety disorders in African Americans* (pp. 203–224). New York: Springer.

Levy, R. H., & Moreland, T. A. (1984). Rationale for monitoring free drug levels. *Clinical Pharmacokinetics, 9*(1), 1–9.

Lidwig, E. G., & Collete, J. (1970). Dependency, social isolation and mental health in a disabled population. *Social Psychiatry, 5,* 92–95.

Lieberman, P. B., & Strauss, J. S. (1984). The recurrence of mania: Environmental factors and medical treatment. *American Journal of Psychiatry, 141,* 77–80.

Lin, K. M. (1987). Experiences on inpatient wards: Taiwan vs. Los Angeles. *American Journal of Social Psychiatry, 7,* 220–225.

Lin, K. M., & Kleinman, A. M. (1988). Psychopathology and clinical course of schizophrenia: A cross-cultural perspective. *Schizophrenia Bulletin, 14,* 555–567.

Lin, K. M., Lau, J. K., Smith, R., & Poland, R. E. (1988). Comparison of alprazolam plasma levels and behavioral effects in normal Asian and Caucasian male volunteers. *Psychopharmacology, 96,* 365–369.

Lin, K. M., & Poland, R. E. (1995). Ethnicity, culture, and psychopharmacology. In F. E. Bloom & D. I. Kupfer (Eds.), *Psychopharmacology: The fourth generation of progress* (pp. 1907–1918). New York: Raven Press.

Lin, K. M., Poland, R. E., Lau, J., & Rubin, R. T. (1988). Haloperidol and prolactin concentrations in Asians and Caucasians. *Journal of Clinical Psychopharmacology, 8,* 195–201.

Lin, K. M., Poland, R. E., & Nakasaki, G. (1993). *Psychopharmacology and psychobiology of ethnicity.* Washington, DC: American Psychiatric Press.

Lin, K. M., Poland, R. E., Nuccio, I., Brammer, G., Zheng, Y., McGeoy, S., Smith, M., & Lesser, I. M. *Ethnicity and imipramine responses: Pharmacokinetic and pharmacogenetic influences.* Manuscript submitted for publication.

Lin, K. M., Poland, R. E., Nuccio, I., Matsuda, K., Hathuc, N., Su, T. P., & Fu, P. (1989). Longitudinal assessment of haloperidol dosage and serum concentration in Asian and Caucasian schizophrenic patients. *American Journal of Psychiatry, 146,* 1307–1311.

Lin, K. M., & Shen, W. W. (1991). Pharmacotherapy for Southeast Asian psychiatric patients. *Journal of Nervous and Mental Disease, 179,* 346–350.

Liu, G. T. (1991). Effects of some compounds isolated from Chinese medicinal herbs on hepatic microsomal cytochrome P-450 and their potential biological consequences. *Drug Metabolism Reviews, 23,* 439–465.

Livingston, R. L., Zucker, D. K., Isenberg, K., & Wetzel, R. D. (1983). Tricyclic antidepressants and delirium. *Journal of Clinical Psychiatry, 44,* 173–176.

Llerena, A., Alm, C., Dahl, K., Ekqvist, B., & Bertilsson, L. (1992). Haloperidol disposition is dependent upon debrisoquine hydroxylation phenotype. *Therapeutic Drug Monitoring, 14,* 92–97.

Marcus, L. R., & Cancro, R. (1982). Pharmacotherapy of Hispanic depressed patients: Clinical observations. *American Journal of Psychotherapy, 36,* 505–512.

Mendoza, R. P., Smith, M. W., Poland, R. E., Lin, K. M., & Strickland, T. L. (1991). Ethnic psychopharmacology: The Hispanic and Native American perspective. *Psychopharmacology Bulletin, 27,* 449–461.

Midha, K. K., Hawes, E. M., Hubbard, J. W., Korchinski, E. D., & McKay, G. (1988a). A pharmacokinetic study of trifluoperazine in two ethnic populations. *Psychopharmacology, 95,* 333–338.

Midha, K. K., Hawes, E. M., Hubbard, J. W., Korchinski, E. D., & McKay G. (1988b). Variation in the single dose pharmacokinetics of fluphenazine in psychiatric patients. *Psychopharmacology, 96,* 206–211.

Moser, M., & Lunn, J. (1981). Comparative effects of pindolol and hydrochlorothiazide in Black hypertensive patients. *Angiology, 32,* 561–566.

Myers, J. K., Lindenthal, J. J., Pepper, M. P., & Ostrander, D. R. (1972). Life events and mental status: A longitudinal study. *Journal of Health and Social Behavior, 13,* 398–406.

Neal, A. M., & Turner, S. M. (1991). Anxiety disorders research with African-Americans: Current status. *Psychological Bulletin, 109,* 400–410.

Nelson, E., Stason, W., Neutra, R., & Solomon, H. S. (1980). Identification of noncompliant hypertensive patients. *Preventive Medicine, 9,* 504–517.

Nemeroff, C. B, DeVane, L., & Pollock, B. G. (1996). Newer antidepressants and the cytochrome P450 system. *American Journal of Psychiatry, 153,* 311–320.

Okpaku, S., Frazer, A., & Mendels, J. (1980). A pilot study of racial differences in erythrocyte lithium transport. *American Journal of Psychiatry, 137,* 120–121.

Pi, E. H., Simpson, G. H., & Cooper, M. A. (1986). Pharmacokinetics of desipramine in Caucasian and Asian volunteers. *American Journal of Psychiatry, 143,* 1174–1176.

Pi, E. H., Tran-Johnson, T. K., Walker, N. R., Cooper, R. B., Suckow, R. F., & Gray, G. E. (1989). Pharmacokinetics of desipramine in Asian and Caucasian volunteers. *Psychopharmacology Bulletin, 25,* 483–487.

Pollock, B. G. (1994). Recent developments in drug metabolism of relevance to psychiatrists. *Harvard Review of Psychiatry, 2,* 204–213.

Potkin, S. G., Shen, Y., Pardes, H., Phelps, B. H., Zhou, D., Shu, L., Korpi, E., & Wyatt, R. J. (1984). Haloperidol concentrations elevated in Chinese patients. *Psychiatry Research, 12,* 167–172.

Preskorn, S. H. (1993). Pharmacokinetics of antidepressants: Why and how they are relevant to treatment. *Journal of Clinical Psychiatry, 54*(Suppl.), 14–34.

Price, N. D., Glazer, W. M., & Morgenstern, H. (1985). Race and the use of fluphenazine decanoate. *American Journal of Psychiatry, 142,* 1491–1492.

Rabkin, J. G., McGrath, P. J., Quitkin, F. M, Tricamo, E., Stewart, J. W., & Klein, D. F. (1990). Effects of pill-giving on maintenance of placebo response in patients with chronic mild depression. *American Journal of Psychiatry, 147,* 1622–1626.

Riesenman, C. (1995). Antidepressant drug interactions and the cytochrome P450 system: A critical appraisal. *Pharmacotherapy, 15*(Suppl.), 84S–99S.

Rudorfer, M. V., Lane, E. A., Chang, W. H., Zhang, M. D., & Potter, W. Z. (1984). Desipramine pharmacokinetics in Chinese and Caucasian volunteers. *British Journal of Clinical Pharmacology, 17,* 433–440.

Rudorfer, M. V., & Robins, E. (1982). Amitriptyline overdose: Clinical effects on tricyclic antidepressant plasma levels. *Journal of Clinical Psychiatry, 43,* 457–460.

Rutledge, D. R., Steinberg, M. B., & Cardozo, L. (1989). Racial differences in drug response: Isoproterenol effects on heart rate following intravenous metoprolol. *Clinical Pharmacology and Therapeutics, 45,* 380–386.

Shader, R. I., & Greenblatt, D. J. (1988). Bees, ginseng and MAOI's revisited. *Journal of Clinical Psychopharmacology, 8,* 325.

Silver, B., Poland, R. E., & Lin, K. M. (1993). Ethnicity and the pharmacology of tricyclic antidepressants. In K. M. Lin, R. E. Poland, & G. Nakasaki (Eds.), *Psychopharmacology and psychobiology of ethnicity* (pp. 61–89). Washington DC: American Psychiatric Press.

Smith, M., Lin, K. M., & Mendoza, R. (1993). "Non-biological" issues affecting psychopharmacotherapy: Cultural considerations. In K. M. Lin, R. E. Poland, & G. Nakasaki (Eds.), *Psychopharmacology and psychobiology of ethnicity* (pp. 37–58). Washington, DC: American Psychiatric Press.

Strickland, T., Lin, K. M., Fu, P., Anderson, D., & Zheng, Y. P. (1995). Comparison of lithium ratio between African-American and Caucasian bipolar patients. *Biological Psychiatry, 37,* 325–330.

Wang, S. L., Huang, J. D., Lai, M. D., Liu, B. H., & Lai, M. L. (1993). Molecular basis of genetic variation in debrisoquine hydroxylation in Chinese subjects: Polymorphism in RFLP and DNA sequence of CYP2D6. *Clinical Pharmacology and Therapeutics, 53,* 410–418.

Weber, W. W. (1987). *The acetylator genes and drug responses.* New York: Oxford University Press.

Westermeyer, J. (1989a). *Psychiatric care of migrants: A clinical guide.* Washington, DC: American Psychiatric Press.

Westermeyer, J. (1989b). *Mental health for refugees and other migrants.* Springfield, IL: Charles C Thomas.

White, L., Tursky, B., & Schwartz, G. E. (Eds.). (1985). *Placebo: Theory, research and mechanisms.* New York: Guilford Press.

Wolff, P. H. (1972). Ethnic differences in alcohol sensitivity. *Science, 175,* 449–450.

Yakota, H., Tamura, S., Furuya, H., Kimura, S., Watanabe, M., Kanazawa, I., Kondo, I., & Gonzalez, F. J. (1993). Evidence for a new variant CYP2D6 allele CY2D6J in a Japanese population associated with lower in vivo rates of sparteine metabolism. *Pharmacogenetics, 3,* 256–263.

Yamashita, I., & Asano, Y. (1979). Tricyclic antidepressants: Therapeutic plasma level. *Psychopharmacology Bulletin, 15,* 40–41.

Yoshida, A. (1993). Genetic polymorphisms of alcohol-metabolizing enzymes related to alcohol sensitivity and alcoholic diseases. In K. M. Lin, R. E. Poland, & G. Nakasaki (Eds.), *Psychopharmacology and psychobiology of ethnicity* (pp. 169–186). Washington, DC: American Psychiatric Press.

Zhang, Y., Reviriego, J., Lou, Y., Sjoqvist, F., & Bertilsson, L. (1990). Diazepam metabolism in native Chinese poor and extensive hydroxylators of S-mephenytoin: Interethnic differences in comparison with white subjects. *Clinical Pharmacology and Therapeutics, 48,* 496–502.

Zhou, H. H., Koshakji, R. P., Siolberstein, D. J., Wilkinson, G. R., & Wood, A. J. J. (1989). Altered sensitivity to and clearance of propranolol in men of Chinese descent as compared with American whites. *New England Journal of Medicine, 320,* 565–570.

Ziegler, V. E., & Biggs, J. T. (1977). Tricyclic plasma levels: Effect of age, race, sex, and smoking. *Journal of the American Medical Association, 438,* 2167–2169.

Zito, J. M., Craig, T. J., Wanderling, J., & Seigel, C. (1987). Pharmaco-epidemiology in 136 hospitalized schizophrenic patients. *American Journal of Psychiatry, 144,* 778–782.

11

Culture and Anxiety: A Clinical and Research Agenda

LAURENCE J. KIRMAYER

With the turn of the millenium just a few years away, anxiety about the future seems only fitting: We live in a world marked by starvation, war, terrorism, and pandemic (Dunant & Porter, 1996). Even economically fortunate countries face the challenges of globalization and "creolization"—the intermixing of different cultures with blurring of boundaries and genres—which bring increased demands for tolerance of complexity, diversity, and living at the edge of chaos (Bibeau, 1997). In the cyberpunk vision of William Gibson we face a near future in which the warmth of the body and the soothing capacity of human connection will be displaced by a global network of electronic communication that creates the virtual world of cyberspace (Gibson, 1996). Solace can be found in virtual communities where fantasies are shared behind masks or with faceless anonymity. The overwhelming message is of a world where the local human scale is threatened by global economic forces and pressures of information exchange that challenge the capacity of any individual to understand and assimilate novelty.

The pervasiveness of anxiety in the modern world seems to make it a problem not so much of the individual as of culture itself and may lead us to view anxiety as normal, expectable, or inevitable. Yet, anxiety is a serious health problem associated with social disability, excess morbidity, and even mortality. Anxiety causes immune suppression, and patients with anxiety disorders may be more susceptible to infectious diseases (Gerritsen, Heinen, Wiegant, Bermond, & Frijda, 1996; La Via et al., 1996). People with panic disorders are at risk for suicide (Weissman, Klerman, Markowitz, & Ouellette, 1989) and—ironically, in the light of the constant reassurances given by mental health practitioners—are also at an increased risk for heart attack (Weissman, Markowitz, Ouellette, Greenwald, & Kahn, 1990).

The challenge for the clinician then is how to situate the problem of anxiety within the larger social and cultural world. In this concluding chapter, I consider the future of research and clinical approaches to anxiety disorders from the perspective of cultural psychiatry. My aim is to identify some emergent issues for research and clinical innovation. In the first section, I will discuss the implications of recent work in emotion theory for the place of culture in emotional experience. The second section briefly reviews evidence for cultural variations in the symptoms and mechanisms of anxiety disorders. The third section reviews some general clinical issues of immediate relevance to practice in ethnically diverse societies. Finally, I consider the broader social context of anxiety disorders and outline an agenda for future research.

VARIETIES OF EMOTIONAL EXPERIENCE

What we call emotion is a complex bodily, cognitive, and social web of experience and behavior. However much they reflect hard-wired motivational systems of adaptive significance, emotions also fold in cultural meanings and practices. Through emotions we are apprised of what matters to us and can signal to others essential information about our own situation and concerns.

The term "emotion" comes from roots meaning *to move*. In folk psychology there is the assumption that emotions move us and that, in some sense, we are not in control of our feelings (Averill, 1972, 1985). Psychologically, this is supported by theories of emotion as subserved by older structures of the brain (the limbic system) (MacLean, 1980) that can react more quickly, impressionistically, and, at times, independently of rational thought (Zajonc, 1984). The passionate heat of emotion then is contrasted with cool reason, and, although emotion has its virtues, rationality and deliberation are not among them.

This theory ignores the sense in which emotions are part of the process and the outcome of social and moral thinking (Harré & Parrott, 1996). Emotions have social and moral significance; indeed, they are a kind of thinking with and through the body about matters of personal and collective significance (Rosaldo, 1984). In a sense then, there is a rationality of emotion (de Sousa, 1987). This affective logic is well suited to figure out the appropriate response to complex social situations, to rationalize a conflict-laden heterarchy of desire, and organize behaviors in terms of salient motives (Damasio, 1994).

Emotions organize behavior into ecologically meaningful patterns, coordinating physical readiness to act (i.e., posture, stance), perception, and memory (Lazarus, 1991). Thus, when fearful, it is useful to be physically ready to flee, to scan the environment for potential threats and escape routes, and to access all that one knows about surviving catastrophes. Many of the internal physiological concomitants of emotion are related to its role in readying the individual for specific forms of action (Cannon, 1929/1963). As experiential reflections of physiological states, emotions highlight personally and socially salient events in the individual's consciousness.

The cognitive functions of emotion in organizing memory lead to the phenomenon of affective state-dependent memory in which knowledge is tied to the mood state in which it was acquired (Bower, 1981). This organization of memory may have adaptive significance because it allows us to partition our knowledge and experience into domains unified by a common motivational or emotional state. Thus, fear mobilizes memories of other fearful occasions, which may yield solutions to our present predicament.

Emotions evolved as part of a system of intraspecies communication and serve to communicate vital information about self and others (Lazarus, 1991). For example, facial expressions of fear signal the threatening nature of a situation to others and may evoke vicarious fear (Hatfield, Cacioppo, & Rapson, 1994). This communicative function of emotion accounts for its intimate links with facial expression (Ekman, 1984). Emotions are thus intrinsically social, and their dynamics are not simply intrapsychic but also interpersonal.

Many authorities on emotion agree there are a few basic emotions tied to motivational states of adaptive significance that are found in some recognizable form around the world (Ekman & Davidson, 1994). In most accounts, these include happiness, sadness, anger, fear, disgust, and surprise. Of course, the cognate emotions in other cultures are not called by the same names and may not have the same connotations or associations. There is no reason—other than ethnocentrism—to assume that the English lexicon provides the best approximation to the underlying categories of emotion. More accurately, the English basic emotion terms represent one cultural configuration of underlying "central motive states" that are configured differently in other cultures (Bindra, 1969). Because all human experience depends on cultural knowledge, including language, gesture, and patterns of interaction, for its realization, there is no basic emotional experience or expression that is free of culture. Nevertheless, whether because they represent pan-human brain states or universal existential predicaments, the core of basic emotions provide a foundation for intercultural communication and empathy on which mutual understanding can be built.

More complex emotions or sentiments are more difficult to translate cross-culturally. In most cases, emotions do not simply name a motivational state or a distinct bodily experience but are names for how one feels in a particular type of situation. The cultural description of this situation involves specific antecedent events, a current disposition to act, and the expected response of others. More complex emotions, then, depend on a broad social context for their meaning and cannot be reduced to brain states or behavioral patterns of an individual. In a sense, emotions name the individual's posture vis-à-vis some larger configuration of the social world, or his or her place in an extended sequence of action and reaction that, by its very expectability (or surprising deviation from what is normatively expected), constitutes the emotion. Developmental experiences and ongoing interactions in this wider social context also inform the private experience of emotion. More publicly, emotions are linked to certain display rules— ways of showing feelings—that are learned throughout childhood and refined across the lifespan. These display rules also shape emotional experience and cognition.

The linguist Anne Wierzbicka (1992) has shown how the meaning of emotion terms in a culture's lexicon can be decomposed into "semantic primitives"—simple statements about actions, positions, and dispositions to respond to circumstances. These statements are sufficiently simple and concrete that they approach universality. For example, the English term *afraid* can be decomposed (p. 133):

> (*X* is) *afraid*
> *X* thinks something like this
>   something bad can happen
>   I don't want this
>   I want to do something because of this
>   I don't know what I can do
> because of this, *X* feels something bad

Wierzbicka's semantic primitives leave unanalyzed the language of evaluation (good/bad), feeling, and desire (want, hope, wish for), which are all based on facts of embodiment as much as linguistic conventions. To assume that her linguistic decompositions provide adequate or complete glosses of the meaning of emotion terms would be to accept an unlikely propositional structure for the representation of emotions. Nevertheless, these decompositions can help us appreciate some important cultural differences.

Complex sentiments can be built up out of simpler feelings and predicaments. Consider, for example the several different types of fear found in the lexicon of the Inuit (Eskimo). In her ethnography of the Utku Inuit of the Canadian Arctic, Jane Briggs (1970) identified four terms related to fear and two to anxiety: *tupak* referred to startle, *kappia* and *iqhi* to fear of physical injury, and *ilira* to fear of being treated unkindly (pp. 343–350). The anxiety terms were less clearly defined in the conversations Briggs took part in but roughly corresponded to different types of apprehension or worry.

These terms make distinctions that are intelligible to English speakers but not basic to our lexicon. Thus, the thought "something bad could happen" characteristic of *afraid*, is replaced in *kappia* by the specific threat of injury, which could come from a natural event, a spiritual force, or a threatening person. In contrast, *ilira* is felt only in relation to people from whom one fears unkind treatment. A child may feel *ilira* toward a stern father. The appropriate response to *ilira* is not to impose on the person, but to obey them or otherwise appease them with friendly gestures. In Wierzbicka's (1992) style of decomposition (though without restricting the vocabulary to her list of semantic primitives):

> (X is) *kappia*
> X thinks something like this
>> I could get injured
>> I don't want this
>> I want to do something because of this
>> I don't know what I can do
> because of this, X feels something bad

A feeling clearly distinct from:

> (X is) *ilira*
> X thinks something like this
>> this person Y may treat me unkindly
>> I don't want this
>> I want to do something because of this
>>> I must be friendly to Y
>>> I must not impose on Y
>>> I must obey Y
> because of this, X feels something bad

This form of semantic analysis allows us to begin to understand another culture's emotion terms from the outside, even as it lays bare the very different connotations and significance of emotions given central place in different cultural systems of meaning. What it obscures is the fact that emotions are not primarily cognitive or semantic structures but ways of knowing that are embodied both in the individual and in patterns and sequences of social interaction with wider cultural meaning. Thus, in the example of *ilira*, the injunctions to be friendly, not to impose, and to obey the feared person may not be conscious thoughts but learned dispositions or stances acquired through modeling and other forms of implicit learning. As well, in Inuit interaction, others may be aware of the feelings of *ilira* that they engender and adjust their own behavior accordingly. In intercultural settings, such responsiveness may be based on misunderstandings. For example, the friendliness of Inuit to strangers may be misinterpreted as indicating more acceptance or affection than is the case.

The fact that emotional behavior, like other cultural phenomena, is acquired through body practices and the implicit learning of procedural knowledge means that people cannot completely describe all the salient features of their own emotional states. This creates a challenge for the clinician: It is not sufficient simply to ask people about their feelings; one must learn through observation (and take advantage of the participant observation of others recorded in ethnographies) to make cultural codes of politeness, interaction, and emotion intelligible.

ANXIETY IN THE MATRIX OF CULTURE

Culture is not so much one factor among many shaping emotion as it is the interactional matrix in which behavior and experience receive meaning. As such, the effects of culture on pathology are not only pathoplastic—shaping symptomatology—but also pathogenic—contributing to the origins and course of psychiatric disorders (Kirmayer, 1989a, 1991). In this section, I briefly consider some ways in which culture influences both the symptoms of anxiety disorders and their underlying mechanisms.

Symptoms of Anxiety

Anxiety disorders commonly overlap with other forms of distress including depressive, dissociative, and somatoform disorders. Cultural differences may increase this overlap, making the identification of discrete anxiety disorders more difficult, if not misleading. For example, the field trials for mixed anxiety–depression in the fourth edition of the *Diagnostic and Statistical Manual of Mental Disorders* (DSM-IV; American Psychiatric Association, 1994) found that 15–20% of Hispanic patients had anxiety disorder not otherwise specified, much of which would fit this pattern of a blurring of depression and anxiety symptoms (Zinbarg et al., 1994). Insisting that patients' symptoms must fit one or other DSM category applies a procrustean bed that leaves out essential elements of their distress. Indeed, the overlap of major classes of disorder ultimately may tell us something important about shared mechanisms rather than simply representing the random co-occurrence of prevalent disorders, as suggested by the term *comorbidity*.

There are many culture-specific symptoms that may be associated with anxiety. For example, in Africa, sensations of worms or parasites crawling in the head are nondelusional expressions of distress (Awaritefe, 1988). In equatorial regions including Africa and Asia, feelings of heat in the head are common nonspecific somatic symptoms (Ebigbo, 1986). Similar symptoms associated with intense emotion have been described among Salvadorean refugees in the United States (Jenkins & Valiente, 1994). Interestingly, when questioned directly, many British medical students also report experiencing "heat in the head," suggesting that some bodily sensations occur across cultures but are not recognized as salient symptoms if they do not fit local categories of distress (Mumford, 1989). In South Asia, many men with anxiety-related problems report loss of semen in the urine, which is both an explanation for debilitation and a cause for worry in itself (Bhatia & Malik, 1991). These culture-related symptoms are not specific to anxiety, being found across the range of mood disorders as well as with adjustment disorders or problems in living that do not reach the threshold for a psychiatric diagnosis. Clinicians unfamiliar with these symptoms may misinterpret them as evidence of physical illness, somatization, or even psychosis, leading to misdiagnosis and inappropriate treatment.

Somatic symptoms are a prominent aspect of most forms of anxiety. People in most cultures commonly attribute the physical symptoms associated with anxiety and panic to bodily illness, a form of somatization (Kirmayer & Robbins, 1991). Such somatic attributions prompt help seeking for medical illness. Patients with panic disorder and generalized anxiety disorder often consult cardiologists with the conviction they have heart disease (Beitman, Mukerji, Flaker, & Basha, 1988; Logue et al., 1993). Other patients consult neurologists for dizziness, paresthesia, headache, or other anxiety-related symptoms. When patients deemphasize the emotional and cognitive aspects of anxiety and view it as entirely secondary to their somatic illness, primary care physicians are less likely to recognize that there is a psychiatric disorder or, indeed, any psychosocial problem (Kirmayer, Robbins, Dworkind, & Yaffe, 1993). Medical specialists may rule out organic illness and dismiss the patient without identifying a treatable anxiety disorder that can account for their symptoms.

The notion of somatization is an expression of Western mind–body dualism. The psychodynamic assumption that somatic and emotional expressions of distress are competing alternatives is not borne out by epidemiological research (Simon & Von Korff, 1991). In fact, most people who are distressed express both somatic and emotional distress, and the two are highly correlated. Most somatic distress is not indicative of a somatization disorder but of the use of a culturally and socially prescribed idiom for expressing distress and for appropriate illness behavior at the doctor's office (Kirmayer & Young, in press). Of course, there is a reluctance on the part of many people—not only Asians and other ethnocultural groups, but the majority of people in North America—to discuss emotional distress or personal problems with a doctor, primarily because of shame and fear of stigmatization. This reluctance finds its mirror in the disinterest of many mental health practitioners in the somatic distress of their patients. Given the salience of somatic symptoms in anxiety disorders, the situation is ripe for misunderstanding.

For example, the Korean syndrome of *hwa-byung*, characterized by anger, anxiety, and depression with a feeling of tightness or a mass in the chest, is less a discrete syndrome than a cultural idiom of distress or an illness explanation consonant with ethnophysiological ideas as well as sociopolitical concerns (Lin et al., 1992). Clinicians unfamiliar with the idiom may misinterpret patients' complaints as indicating physical illness and miss the personal and social basis of symptoms when this is taken for granted or suppressed by patients.

Anxiety itself may constitute a cultural idiom. In many parts of Central America, *susto*—illness caused by fright—is an important etiological category that links shocking or startling personal events to the gamut of health conditions (Rubel, O'Nell, & Collado-Ardn, 1984). Fright is thought to cause infection, fever, and death or, when it affects a pregnant woman, may result in birth defects. This conventional use of fear as a causal explanation for illness and misfortune has little or no correlation with individual psychopathology or anxiety disorders; it serves instead to link personal distress to environmental circumstances in a way that is locally intelligible and that justifies subsequent illness and disability (Holloway, 1994).

Similarly, the notion of "nerves" is common in many cultures as an idiom of distress for talking about a wide range of physical and emotional symptoms, worries, and social concerns (Low, 1994). Like the idiom of stress, talk about "nerves" tends to diffuse the sources and personal meanings of troubles, although it also conveys some sense of individual vulnerability or sensitivity. Often, however, this individual psychological vulnerability is downplayed, while links between social problems or stresses and somatic distress are emphasized in a form of sociosomatic theory. The idiom of nerves provides a way to map out problems in the social domain using the nervous system as a sort of "dowsing rod." Talk about nerves and nervousness here is both a reflection of predicaments and an effort to position oneself. Sociosomatics is both an empirical model of causation and a cultural concept linked to broader ideologies of the person. Symptoms, then, are not just manifestations of illness but also signs or tokens in a larger semiotic game.

Mechanisms of Anxiety

The cognitive theory of anxiety emphasizes the loop between bodily feelings of distress and catastrophizing thoughts (Clark et al., 1988). This cognitive loop includes interpretations of bodily sensations as symptoms (attributing them to illness or to emotion that is pathological in its form or intensity), evaluations of perceived threat and ability to cope, and anticipation of the responses of others (Salkovskis, 1989). Self-labeling of emotion as pathological and oneself as "out of control" may contribute to emotional distress and disability (Thoits, 1985).

There is a growing body of work in discursive psychology that shows how persons and selves are constructed through conversation and narration with others (Bruner, 1990; Harré & Gillett, 1994). Particular forms of self-narration and discursive practices may contribute to psychopathology. For example, the hallmark of agoraphobia is "the attempt to exert control over a highly circumscribed space, to create a safe haven within a chaotic, often unwelcoming universe" (Capps & Ochs, 1995, p. 3). Close analysis of the discourse of one woman suffering from panic disorder with agoraphobia revealed the ways in which her own recollection and retelling of her illness helped to consolidate her fear and disability: "Meg casts anxiety as a force that acts upon her. Meg deputizes her sensations as the creative subject and becomes a passive destination for their catastrophic energy" (p. 69). Her accounts of her illness "prolong the narrative reconstruction of panic experiences as a focal point of current consciousness" (p. 65).

Narrative accounts of the self in illness and health are shaped by cultural conceptions of the person (Howard, 1991). Cultural differences in the concept of the person result in different standards for self-control and self-efficacy, and different demands for cognitive or behavioral consistency (Markus & Kitayama, 1991). Folk psychological notions about control provide the standards against which the person (and significant others) can judge their behavior as normal and expectable or pathologically out of control. The illness narratives of people with anxiety disorders reveal a rich vocabulary expressing gradations of loss of control (Capps & Ochs, 1995, p. 66). The same cultural notions about control help to make certain forms of anxiety more prevalent. If what escapes from personal control is viewed as the normal, expectable workings of fate, God, or happenstance, and no added effort at reestablishing self-control is mandated, then the person may feel relatively little anxiety. If social expectations are such that tight control over one's behavior is expected in a specific context, then even minor failures or deviations from norms may result in significant anxiety and lead to escalating cycles of emotional distress. Something like this has been proposed to explain the relatively high prevalence of social phobias in Japan and Korea (Kirmayer, 1991).

Taijin kyofusho is a common form of social phobia in Japan, characterized by anxiety about public self-presentation and performance but also by the more culture-specific concern that one's inappropriate social behavior—especially inappropriate gaze or staring—will make others uncomfortable. Other symptoms of *taijin kyofusho* include the fear that one has an unpleasant odor or ugly appearance that will also give offense (symptoms of body dysmorphic disorder in DSM-IV). This emphasis on causing discomfort in others reflects the importance given in Japan to harmonious interaction in a complex status hierarchy. Japanese child rearing encourages public and private self-consciousness as ways of regulating behavior. As a result, the symptoms of *taijin kyofusho* may reach delusional intensity, yet perhaps be less indicative of severe pathology than they would be elsewhere; even delusional cases of *taijin kyofusho* often respond to cognitive-behavioral and group psychotherapeutic interventions, including the indigenous Morita therapy.

Clearly, sociocultural factors can reinforce cognitive and interpersonal processes that give rise to anxiety. Cultural factors also influence clinicians' own categories. For example, social phobia was recognized as an important neurosis in Japan in the 1920s, linked closely to neurasthenia and hypochondriasis, whereas it was relatively neglected in U.S. psychiatric nosology until the 1980s, when it was recognized as a cause of serious disability. The World Health Organization cross-national study of psychological problems in general health care revealed that social phobia is a common and disabling condition among patients in primary care that is often unrecognized by physicians (Weiller, Bisserbe, Boyer, Lepine, & Lecrubier, 1996).

The Matrix of Culture

To illustrate further how cultural, social, and cognitive psychological factors interact in a specific instance, consider the cultural idiom of *ataques de nervios*, which has been extensively discussed elsewhere in this volume (see Chapters 1 and 4). Associated with anxiety, anger, emotional shock, and other distressing circumstances, the most common symptoms of *ataques* are "screaming uncontrollably" and attacks of crying; other common symptoms include shouting, expressions of anger, loss of consciousness and amnesia for the episodes (Guarnaccia, Rivera, Franco, Neighbors & Allende-Ramos, 1996). Pathbreaking work by Peter Guarnaccia (Chapter 1, this volume), Roberto Lewis-Fernandez, and others has helped us to understand the social and cultural embedding of *ataques* in Puerto Rican culture.

The idiom of *ataques* is related to broader cultural concerns with gender roles, the political autonomy of Puerto Rico, and the pervasive influences of multinational corporations in manipulating local images of identity. The cultural ideology of *machismo* with its polarization and complementarity of gender roles creates concerns in men about displays of emotion or lack of control as indicating feminization while sanctioning such displays by women. At the same time, the ambivalent relationship of Puerto Rico to the mainland United States contributes to a broader sense of being relatively powerless or "out of control." All of these social forces help to open up a psychological space in which the individual who is frightened, angry, or simply vexed beyond endurance can "let go" to feelings and behaviors of shouting, crying, and otherwise displaying and declaring their loss of control. A personal loss of control is thus made possible not only by a specific cultural model of distress but by larger social forces that reinforce the theme of powerlessness; but here, as in other culturally shaped phenomena, the consciousness and choice of the individual still play a crucial role (Cohen, 1994). In his study of the illness narratives of patients with *ataques*, Lewis-Fernandez (1995) found that some people told of a moment of decision during the *ataques* when they recognized what was happening and decided to "go with it."

This cultural exegesis of *ataques* illustrates the hierarchical embedding of illness experience and cognition. We should not make too much of this specificity, because *ataques* are also common in other Caribbean and Central and South American countries. However, this geographical distribution may also reflect cultural and social continuities across the region.

The loss of control of *ataques* may not be socially sanctioned, in that it still has negative value attached to it, but it exists as a cultural form. Not all culturally shaped behavior is positive, adaptive, sanctioned, or strategically advantageous for individuals or institutions. As Guarnaccia notes (Chapter 1, this volume), some people who have symptoms consistent with an *ataque* prefer to call their problem *nervios* because it implies less loss of control. It is not labeling per se that causes the initial *ataque*; the self-labeling of distress as an *ataque* is part of a cognitive process in which further loss of self-control becomes expectable. As such, what appears locally as chaotic and desperate, seen in a larger context, appears culturally patterned and predictable. In this example, we can see the cultural scripting of self-control. This cultural scripting may extend beyond the dramatic display of emotion in the acute *ataque* to include subsequent dissociative symptoms. Elsewhere, I have tried to show how similar processes, including narrative conventions, cultural models of memory, and occasions for recollection and retelling can shape dissociative experience (Kirmayer, 1994, 1996b).

CLINICAL IMPLICATIONS
OF A CULTURAL PERSPECTIVE

An effort was made in DSM-IV to incorporate information on cultural variations in symptomatology, although the basic structure of criteria remains largely unchanged. The most important addition is the guidelines for the cultural formulation in Appendix I (American Psychiatric Association, 1994). The accompanying glossary of culture-bound syndromes is misleading but may be of some use, if clinicians recognize that most of what is described there are cultural idioms of distress rather than syndromes, that is, flexible ways of talking about a wide range of problems and predicaments that may influence illness experience but that often do not reflect consistent intercorrelations of specific symptoms.

The cultural formulation should become a routine part of the assessment in every case where cultural difference is salient. In outline, a cultural formulation consists of (1) the cultural identity of the patient including reference group(s), language, spiritual/religious affiliation, and multicultural identity; (2) cultural explanations of the illness (i.e., idioms of distress, explanatory models, experience with popular and professional sources of care); (3) cultural factors related to the psychosocial environment and functioning (e.g., cultural influences on stressors, social support, and stigmatization); (4) cultural aspects of the relationship between patient and clinician (e.g., attitudes toward clinical authority, dependency, influence on transference and countertransference); and (5) an overall formulation, synthesizing the above information.

Ethnic and cultural identity have proved to be more important than assumed by the assimilationist ideology of the "melting pot." Acculturation is not equivalent to assimilation. There are many alternative ways to adapt to migration and many immigrants maintain strong affiliations and commitments to both their culture of origin and their new home (Berry, Kim, Power, Young, & Bujaki, 1989). Bilingualism, biculturalism, and other modes of creolization are common and may, in fact, be associated with better mental health than simply jettisoning one's heritage culture for that of the dominant ethnocultural group (Berry, 1988). The fact that people adhere to traditional ideas or have multiple alternative accounts available to them to explain and respond to problems may become particularly important in times of illness. Ambiguities of identity due to migration, culture change, and conflict, as well as the fracture of families and communities, may be sources of anxiety that are worked out in culture-specific terms (Harris, Blue, & Griffith, 1995). In some cases, affliction itself may serve to establish and reinforce one's ethnic identity (Lock, 1990).

Cultural understandings of illness include idioms of distress, explanatory models (Kleinman, 1988), prototypes, and less systematized forms of knowledge (Kirmayer, Young, & Robbins, 1994). Folk illnesses cannot be mapped one to one onto the DSM-IV framework because, in most cases, they represent ways of understanding and categorizing distress that are independent of (orthogonal to) the DSM nosology. The typical folk category cuts across many different DSM diagnoses and has its own network of meanings with psychological and social consequences.

Both the psychiatric diagnosis and the folk label are important, but the cultural formulation must go beyond labels to situate a person's problems in social and cultural context. This larger social context includes family and other relationships that are the source of both stresses and support. In some cases, the individual who presents with anxiety is a barometer of interactional problems within the family system. The identification of systemic problems depends on knowledge about cultural variations in family structure and process across the life cycle (McGoldrick, Giordano, & Pearce, 1996). In many cultures, anxiety may be stigmatized as a loss of emotional control with negative implications for the social standing of the individual and his or her family. Where talk of nerves and worries is accepted as an idiom of distress, anxiety may be inadvertently encouraged and patients may be reluctant to lose its communicative functions.

The clinician–patient relationship is shaped by expectations about the healer's role and the nature of help, and by the position of the clinician in the community. Elements of position include the clinician's's ethnocultural identity, socioeconomic status, and administrative or political authority. Some patients come from traditions where healers are authority figures who are expected to understand the problem without much questioning or divagation and to give clear directives for treatment. Many clinicians are ambivalent about power and prefer to shift responsibility for treatment to the patient. Even a model of collaboration or negotiation may already imply an abdication of clinical authority for some patients, albeit a necessary one both for ethical reasons and as part of larger therapeutic goals of consciousness raising and empowerment.

Much psychotherapy is based on a cultural ideology of individualism that aims for autonomy (Kirmayer, 1989b). Thus, therapy is time limited and the goal is "termination" of the therapeutic relationship. This parallels a model of psychological development in which the transition from adolescence to adulthood involves separation from, and a degree of renunciation of, one's family of origin. In many parts of the world, people expect to remain an integral part of their family of origin or a local tightly knit community throughout their lifespan. Accordingly, relationships with helpers may also be longstanding with no expectation for a complete end to treatment or support. Clearly, these are important issues to explore for patients with anxiety disorders.

The synthesis of information in a cultural formulation may lead to modifications or qualifications of the DSM diagnosis. Ultimately, however, a useful formulation is directed not toward cataloging pathology but toward identifying solutions. Cultural information can be used to select treatment strategies with greater specificity; to adapt existing treatments to the particular needs, resources, and expectations of the patient, and most creatively, to devise new, culturally based approaches (Chin, De La Cancela, & Jenkins, 1993; Kareem & Littlewood, 1992; Vargas & Koss-Chioino, 1992).

The recognition of this need for a shared cultural reality, as well as pragmatic issues of language and accessibility, have prompted the development of ethnospecific services. These services attempt to match clients to appropriate resources. In the context of mental health, ethnic matching can occur at the level of treatment, practitioner, or institution.

Treatment

There are many culture-specific treatments that may help to resolve anxiety problems. Some are closely tied to particular cultural ideologies and practices and so are difficult to learn or practice outside their original context. Others are more easily translated across borders. For example, Morita therapy, a form of cognitive-behavioral, mileu, and group therapy designed in the 1920s by the Japanese psychiatrist Shoma Morita to treat individuals with *shinkeishitsu* (nervous weakness) and *taijin kyofusho* (social phobia), has been adapted and promoted as an effective treatment program for individuals with social phobia, death anxiety, and other forms of anxiety (Ishiyama, 1986; Kitanishi, 1990; Reynolds & Kiefer, 1977).

Meditative practices derived from Buddhism and yogic traditions also are culturally adaptable and have direct applications to the treatment of anxiety. The effectiveness of mindfulness mediation for generalized anxiety disorder and panic disorder indicates the value for individuals from European American cultural backgrounds of the psychological insights of Theravada Buddhism even when divorced from part of their larger religious context (Miller, Fletcher, & Kabat-Zinn, 1995).

The religious context and system of meaning itself is an important resource for patients who accept and participate in these practices. Religious meanings and sources of support can be found by working with members of the community. The family therapist Melissa Griffith (1995) has shown the power of encouraging Christian patients to have private conversations with God, as a way of invoking transcendent integrative functions when personal and family quandaries seem insoluble.

Alternative or complementary medicine provides a range of useful techniques for managing tension and anxiety that can be useful adjuncts to conventional mental health care and that are finding increasingly wide acceptance in North America. Use of these practices is not restricted to one's own tradition; in a study of help seeking in an urban multicultural neighborhood we found frequent borrowing of types of care across cultural boundaries (Kirmayer, Young, Galbaud du Fort, Weinfeld, & Lasry, 1996). Clinicians' interest in and willingness to work with these other resources will encourage patients to take a more active part in their own care.

Practitioners

The availability of professionals from the same cultural background as the client sends an implicit message of acceptance and understanding. Of course, the mere presence of a minority clinician, although it may contribute to patients' self-esteem through identification with a successful compatriot, is no guarantee that the individual patient will be understood. Clinicians with inside knowledge may still benefit from training in anthropology and other social sciences to help them integrate their cultural knowledge with professional perspectives, without either rejecting their background or overgeneralizing from their own, sometimes idiosyncratic experience. If the clinician offers only conventional treatment with little attempt to understand or adapt to the client's specific cultural beliefs, then the match is more in appearance than reality.

Where clinicians from the same background as the patient are not available, culture brokers and interpreters who are trained and integrated into the mental health team may provide some of the same benefits. Consultation and collaboration with healers and religious leaders from the patient's community or tradition can provide important ideas, sanctioning of treatment, and leverage for change. The introduction of an interpreter or culture broker, and the use of community consultants, are systemic interventions, and potential coalitions and conflicts of interest must be carefully considered. As well, work with religious practitioners or alternative healers can raise ethical issues due to differences in values and epistemologies. These must be openly acknowledged and negotiated with respect for the client's own cultural background and in accordance with the clinician's professional ethics and personal limits of tolerance.

Institutions

In some cases, specific services have been set up at an institutional level to concentrate the requisite linguistic, cultural and clinical expertise to provide services to ethnocultural communities. An institution run by and for a cultural community is likely to receive greater trust and acceptance. Other clinics have identified themselves as specially aligned with antiracist or other political stances that make them more acceptable to oppressed minorities (Kareem & Littlewood, 1992). For small communities, however, ethnospecific clinics may actually be disadvantageous, because patients are likely to bump into friends and acquaintances from within the community and the privacy and anonymity sought for in professional mental health cannot be maintained.

The great cultural diversity in many North American cities, and increasingly limited health care resources, also work against the development of ethnospecific services. As a result, there is a need for all clinicians to develop a basic level of generic cultural competence and to supplement this with more detailed knowledge of those groups with whom they do most of their work. To do this, we need information about the range and modal patterns of behavior of an ethnocultural group. The paradox is that culture is first and foremost about historical particulars but cultural competence must involve some general and generalizable skills. Too often, this is translated into learning about coarse cultural stereotypes, which are intended to guide the clinician.

The cultural formulation provides one way to deal with the problem of stereotyping cultural groups. By focusing on the minute particulars of a case—and, over the course of training, seeing many cases—clinicians will develop a more differentiated model and the skills to reformulate each case anew. As such, the cultural formulation works against the homogenizing effects of both diagnostic categories and cultural stereotypes.

What does generic cultural competence consist of and how can it be achieved? The culturally competent clinician will do the following:

1. Approach each case as unique and individual, but focus on the social and cultural context of the behavior and experience of the identified patient and his or her family; emphasize knowledge of culture, language, and etiquette as modes of inquiry rather than as *a priori* answers to the dilemmas of a specific case.
2. Understand the range of variation in a cultural group and its significance for individuals and the group; in this way, recognize when culture is camouflage for problems at other levels and when it is constitutive.
3. Be able to formulate cultural dynamics as part of a comprehensive processual model of pathology and design interventions to address the most flexible or accessible level of the individual, family, or social system.

Pedagogical strategies to achieve cultural competence in trainees follow directly from these goals: (1) Emphasize the method of inquiry rather than the specific cultural information that emerges in a given case; (2) present many different cases, giving a sense of the wide range of variation; and (3) emphasize processes or links between social, psychological, and physiological events so that what is learned is a deeper structure of the mediation between individual experience and psychopathology and social and systemic factors. Specific cultural themes (e.g., styles of emotional expression or containment, modes of family life, central values) take on their clinical significance in the context of these more detailed models.

A RESEARCH AGENDA

At present, cognitive theories offer the easiest way to understand the impact of culture on anxiety. Future research may well identify ethnocultural and temperamental differences in the biology of anxiety linked to variations in lifestyle, diet, environment and genome. The work of Keh-Ming Lin and colleagues (see Chapter 10, this volume) on ethnocultural variations in drug metabolism illustrates this link with biology. Notwithstanding the current emphasis within psychiatry on biological theories and pharmacological interventions, however, future research must focus on the interplay among physiological, psychological, and social processes.

Epidemiological studies must canvas culture-specific symptoms if they are to arrive at meaningful estimates of prevalence and adequate characterization of the problems in a community. Beyond simply counting the prevalence of problems, substantive epidemiology should include social and cultural indicators that could help explain observed differences. In particular, measures of disability and outcome can help validate diagnostic categories and folk labels as clinically relevant.

Somatic and dissociative symptoms are important cross-culturally and are given insufficient emphasis in the DSM-IV characterization of anxiety disorders, with both too few and too narrow a range of symptoms represented. This symptom variation, and the overlap among anxiety, depressive, somatoform, and dissociative disorders, raises questions about the most appropriate diagnostic categories and criteria. For example, in the Puerto Rican disaster study, *ataques de nervios* cut across other psychiatric diagnoses (Guarnaccia, Canino, Rubio-Stipec, & Bravo, 1993). The next step in research is to determine the best predictors of illness course, disability, and outcome. Studies using alternative diagnostic criteria incorporating culture-specific items and modified thresholds can identify the most useful nosological scheme to guide assessment of prognosis and prescription of treatment. If the emic (indigenous) category adds additional predictive value beyond the DSM category, or even performs better at predicting acceptance of and response to specific treatments, it should not be viewed as cultural "window dressing" that obscures the essential problem and/or simply can be mapped onto the correct DSM diagnosis.

Recent psychiatric research has emphasized the role of traumatic experiences in childhood or later as etiological factors in a wide range of disorders. Specific types of trauma may predispose to different types of psychopathology, particularly in interaction with premorbid personality traits. The construct of posttraumatic stress disorder has been extended to cover much of the distress that follows catastrophic events. Very high rates of posttraumatic stress disorder have been found in many places in the world where people have endured political violence, terror, and torture (de Girolamo & McFarlane, 1996; Desjarlais, Eisenberg, Good, & Kleinman, 1995, pp. 47–50). This is reflected in the problems of refugee populations in the United States. However, the criteria for posttraumatic stress disorder in the DSM may not put enough emphasis on the importance of dissociative and somatoform symptoms in the experience of many patients worldwide (Kirmayer, 1996a).

Much theorizing about posttraumatic stress disorder treats the link between trauma and subsequent anxiety as a matter of conditioned emotional responses that engrave distressing memories and emotional reactivity on the nervous system. This ignores the sense in which it is less the traumatic event than its personal and social meaning that makes it anxiogenic and more broadly toxic. Many people exposed to life-threatening events have experienced loss as well as trauma and, in their efforts to survive, have been catapulted into a new world that presents a multitude of challenges and dislocations with their own burden of disappointment, frustration, and loss.

A simple arc from traumatic cause to posttraumatic effect is insufficient to understand or help with the problems of displacement, flight, and resettlement. There is evidence that the welfare of refugees depends not only on the trauma and privations they have suffered before and during migration but even more on the outcome of their resettlement in a host country. Migration can lead to suspended or broken narratives of self that contribute to depression and despair due to lack of ability to imagine a safe future, and to anxiety due to a lack of closure, completeness, or coherence. Thinking of migration as a trajectory encourages us to focus on the postmigration situation and the narrative reconstruction of past history rather than simply viewing premigration traumas as the determinants of subsequent adjustment. For example, Eisenbruch (1991) has suggested approaching the predicament of Cambodian refugees—who experienced an unprecedented period of "autogenocide"—in terms of "cultural bereavement" rather than the narrower concept of posttraumatic stress disorder. Such an approach may lead to innovative treatments focussed not just on refugees' biomedical condition or psychiatric diagnosis but on the trajectory their lives follow over the course of migration.

The metaphor of trauma was borrowed from the study of physical injury and surgery (Young, 1995). As such it puts emphasis on the intensity of the traumatic event as a determinant of the degree of psychic "damage." The analogy breaks down quickly in situations where threats to the integrity of the self are prolonged and insidious. It is the social and personal meaning of events that makes them anxiogenic. Events that are not time-limited traumas but persistent sources of worry may lead to more pervasive anxiety.

As an example of historical events, poorly conceptualized as a discrete trauma and, yet, seemingly liable to cause anxiety consider the predicament of African Americans, who still struggle to escape the legacy of slavery (Allen, 1996). Even those who are economically and professionally successful against considerable odds, having "arrived," may feel cheated of peace of mind and security due to the enduring inequities of a racist society (Cose, 1993). The personal experience and impact of these inequities is a source of both anger and anxiety. But where the overriding sense is one of powerlessness and hopelessness, the response may be more of numbing, apathy, and withdrawal than overt anxiety (West, 1993). Posttraumatic stress disorder seems a very pale way to capture the significance of the historical losses and injuries suffered by African Americans or, for that matter, Native Americans (Manson et al., 1996; Robin, Chester & Goldman, 1996)—the more so because structural inequalities and discrimination continue to challenge their lives.

Major events "traumatize" individuals, but the effects are not simply or even primarily inscribed on their nervous system; they are transformed into a social landscape of fear. Families who have had members "disappear" may suffer both unresolvable grief and anxiety due to the open-ended nature of such ambiguous loss. Cultural bereavement is an example of a more encompassing way to conceptualize the impact of trauma that takes into account the temporal trajectory and social embedding of illness experience. The diagnosis of posttraumatic stress disorder falsely homogenizes patients by emphasizing certain physiological, psychological, and sociomoral elements that may, in fact, not be the central issues for many individuals (Young, 1995).

Cultural norms for emotional expression and containment influence the concealment and disclosure, suppression and expression of both traumatic events and emotional reactions including anxiety (Wellenkamp, 1995; Wikan, 1990). Many cultures value emotional containment, equanimity, and the acceptance of suffering as marks of maturity. These same cultural norms and ideologies in turn influence the ability to construct and stabilize a narrative account of one's suffering and current predicament, which may have healing effects. This poses important therapeutic questions as to whether, when, and where patients should be encouraged to disclose and narrate their histories of trauma and distress.

Illness narratives are told with the collaboration of others. Their significance can be understood, not only in intrapsychic terms, but also in terms of this positioning and affiliation vis-à-vis others; the trade-offs they entail can also be understood in these terms. Attempts to act "normal" may aggravate rather than alleviate distress if acting normal means denying the origins or otherwise contributing to a pervasive silencing of the sufferer (Capps & Ochs, 1995, p. 112). In other situations, declarations of loss of control or of abuse may damage relationships vital for one's self-worth as a family member, cause loss of face before the community, or even threaten survival.

CONCLUSION

The multicultural nature of contemporary urban societies has forced a shift in perspective from culture as a homogeneous and homeostatic system of beliefs and practices that fit an "ecological niche," toward the notion of culture as a historical system of knowledge and practice, riven by contradiction and contestation and held together not by conformity or utility but by active participation and exchange. Cultural systems are capable of endless variation and undergo ceaseless change as each individual struggles to make his or her way in the world. This shift in perspective has led to a corresponding shift in the attitudes of cultural psychiatry away from the exotic butterfly collecting of "culture-bound syndromes" and toward the notion of cultural idioms of distress. These idioms are not diagnostic categories and cannot be mapped one to one onto the categories of DSM-IV. They are languages of distress, of self-understanding and communication to others about what troubles and concerns the individual. As such, they are used flexibly, creatively, and, at times, idiosyncratically.

The cognitive theory of anxiety suggests that cultural beliefs, attributions, illness schemas, and broader concepts of mind, self, and person can take part in vicious circles of catastrophizing thoughts, exaggerated feelings of vulnerability and perceived threat, and other attitudes and behaviors that contribute to sustained anxiety. On the other hand, some culturally mediated cognitions may contribute to a sense of security, calm, self-soothing, and equanimity and may support effective coping strategies. Trying to teach a patient a new cognitive or behavioral strategy for coping generally works better if it fits with what is already known or builds on some area of competence that is both well learned and well integrated with other important beliefs, values, and practices, and is likely to be accepted, understood, and reinforced by others.

This last points to the importance of interpersonal interaction in the genesis, course, and treatment of anxiety disorders. Anxiety disorders should not be conceived of as entirely within the skin of the individual. Like all psychological phenomena, they take part in networks of interpersonal interaction that are embedded in larger social structures. The whole is sustained by cultural knowledge and practice. Culturally responsive treatment is based on assessment of this wider social network, which can then be mobilized through family and other social interventions.

In many cases, somatic and psychological symptoms associated with anxiety also function as part of cultural idioms of distress, which are employed to understand and talk about personal conflicts and social predicaments. Lack of familiarity with these idioms may lead to misdiagnosis—overdiagnosing pathology where none is present or missing important problems. At the same time, the cultural idiom offers a language rich with metaphors that may be employed by the clinician to negotiate treatment and to devise cognitive or strategic interventions that reframe patients' experience and lead to better coping and more adaptive behavior.

REFERENCES

Allen, I. M. (1996). PTSD among African Americans. In A. J. Marsella, M. J. Friedman, E. T. Gerrity, & R. M. Scurfield (Eds.), *Ethnocultural aspects of posttraumatic stress disorders: Issues, research and clinical applications* (pp. 209–238). Washington, DC: American Psychological Association.

American Psychiatric Association. (1994). *Diagnostic and statistical manual of mental disorders* (4th ed.). Washington, DC: Author.

Averill, J. R. (1972). An analysis of psychophysiological symbolism and its influence on theories of emotion. *Journal of the Theory of Social Behaviour, 4*(2), 147–190.

Averill, J. R. (1985). The social construction of emotion: With special reference to love. In K. J. Gergen & K. E. Davis (Eds.), *The social construction of the person* (pp. 89–109). New York: Springer-Verlag.

Awaritefe, A. (1988). Clinical anxiety in Nigeria. *Acta Psychiatrica Scandinavica, 77,* 729–735.

Beitman, B. D., Mukerji, V., Flaker, G., & Basha, I. M. (1988). Panic disorder, cardiology patients, and atypical chest pain. *Psychiatric Clinics of North America, 11*(2), 387–397.

Berry, J. W. (1988). Acculturation and mental health. In P. Dasen, J. W. Berry, & N. Sartorius (Eds.), *Health and cross-cultural psychology.* London: Sage.

Berry, J. W., Kim, U., Power, S., Young, M., & Bujaki, M. (1989). Acculturation attitudes in plural societies. *International Review of Applied Psychology, 38,* 185–206.

Bhatia, M. S., & Malik, S. C. (1991). Dhat syndrome: A useful diagnostic entity in Indian culture. *British Journal of Psychiatry, 159,* 691–695.

Bibeau, G. (1997). Cultural psychiatry in a creolizing world: Questions for a new research agenda. *Transcultural Psychiatry, 34*(1), 9–41.

Bindra, D. (1969). A unified interpretation of emotion and motivation. *Annals of the New York Academy of Sciences, 159,* 1071–1083.

Bower, G. H. (1981). Mood and memory. *American Psychologist, 36*(2), 129–148.

Briggs, J. L. (1970). *Never in anger: Portrait of an Eskimo family.* Cambridge, MA: Harvard University Press.

Bruner, J. (1990). *Acts of meaning.* Cambridge, MA: Harvard University Press.

Cannon, W. B. (1963). *Bodily changes in pain, hunger, fear and rage.* New York: Harper & Row. (Original work published 1929)

Capps, L., & Ochs, E. (1995). *Constructing panic: The discourse of agoraphobia.* Cambridge, MA: Harvard University Press.

Chin, J. L., De La Cancela, V., & Jenkins, Y. M. (1993). *Diversity in psychotherapy: The politics of race, ethnicity, and gender.* Westport, CN: Praeger.

Clark, D. M., Salkovskis, P. M., Gelder, M., Koehler, C., Martin, M., Anastasiades, P., Hackmann, A., Middleton, H., & Jeavons, A. (1988). Tests of a cognitive theory of panic. In I. Hand & H. U. Wittchen (Eds.), *Panic and phobias* (Vol. 2, pp. 149–158). Berlin: Springer-Verlag.

Cohen, A. P. (1994). *Self consciousness: An alternative anthropology of identity.* London: Routledge.

Cose, E. (1993). *The rage of a privileged class.* New York: HarperCollins.

Damasio, A. R. (1994). *Descartes' error: Emotion, reason, and the human brain.* New York: G.P. Putnam's Sons.

de Girolamo, G., & McFarlane, A. C. (1996). The epidemiology of PTSD: A comprehensive review of the international literature. In A. J. Marsella, M. J. Friedman, E. T. Gerrity, & R. M. Scurfield (Eds.), *Ethnocultural aspects of posttraumatic stress disorders: Issues, research and clinical applications* (pp. 33–86). Washington, DC: American Psychological Association.

Desjarlais, R., Eisenberg, L., Good, B., & Kleinman, A. (1995). *World mental health: Problems and priorities in low-income countries.* New York: Oxford University Press.

de Sousa, R. (1987). *The rationality of emotion.* Cambridge, MA: MIT Press.

Dunant, S., & Porter, R. (Eds.). (1996). *The age of anxiety.* London: Little, Brown.

Ebigbo, P. O. (1986). A cross-sectional study of somatic complaints of Nigerian females using the Enugu somatization scale. *Culture, Medicine, and Psychiatry, 10*(2), 167–186.

Eisenbruch, M. (1991). From postraumatic stress disorder to cultural bereavement: Diagnosis of Southeast Asian refugees. *Social Science and Medicine, 33*(6), 673–680.

Ekman, P. (1984). Expression and the nature of emotion. In K. Scherer & P. Ekman (Eds.), *Approaches to emotion* (pp. 319–343). Hillsdale, NJ: Erlbaum.

Ekman, P., & Davidson, R. J. (Eds.). (1994). *The nature of emotion: Fundamental questions.* New York: Oxford University Press.

Gerritsen, W., Heinen, C. J., Wiegant, V. M., Bermond, B., & Frijda, N. (1996). Experimental social fear: Immunological, hormonal, and autonomic concomitants. *Psychosomatic Medicine, 58,* 273–286.

Gibson, W. (1996). *Idoru.* New York: G. P. Putnam's Sons.

Griffith, M. E. (1995). Opening therapy to conversations with a personal God. In K. Weingarten (Ed.), *Cultural resistance: Challenging beliefs about men, women, and therapy* (pp. 123–139). New York: Haworth Press.

Guarnaccia, P. J., Canino, G., Rubio-Stipec, M., & Bravo, M. (1993). The prevalence of ataques de nervios in the Puerto Rico disaster study: The role of culture in psychiatric epidemiology. *Journal of Nervous and Mental Disease, 181*(3), 157–165.

Guarnaccia, P. J., Rivera, M., Franco, F., Neighbors, C., & Allende-Ramos, C. (1996). The experiences of *ataques de nervios*: Towards an anthropology of emotions in Puerto Rico. *Culture, Medicine and Psychiatry, 20*(3), 343–367.

Harré, R., & Gillett, G. (1994). *The discursive mind.* Thousand Oaks, CA: Sage.

Harré, R., & Parrott, W. G. (Eds.). (1996). *The emotions: Social, cultural and biological dimensions.* London: Sage.

Harris, H. W., Blue, H. C., & Griffith, E. E. H. (Eds.). (1995). *Racial and ethnic identity: Psychological development and creative expression.* New York: Routledge.

Hatfield, E., Cacioppo, J. T., & Rapson, R. L. (1994). *Emotional contagion.* New York: Cambridge University Press.

Holloway, G. (1994). Susto and the career path of the victim of an industrial accident: A sociological case study. *Social Science and Medicine, 38*(7), 989–997.

Howard, G. S. (1991). Culture tales: A narrative approach to thinking, cross-cultural psychology, and psychotherapy. *American Psychologist, 46*(3), 187–197.

Ishiyama, F. I. (1986). Positive reinterpretation of fear of death: A Japanese (Morita) psychotherapy approach to anxiety treatment. *Psychotherapy, 23*(4), 556–381.

Jenkins, J., & Valiente, M. (1994). Bodily transactions of the passions: El calor among Salvadorean refugees. In T. Csordas (Ed.), *Embodiment and experience: The existential ground of culture and self* (pp. 163–182). New York: Cambridge University Press.

Kareem, J., & Littlewood, R. (Eds.). (1992). *Intercultural therapy: Themes, interpretations and practice.* Oxford: Blackwell Scientific.

Kirmayer, L. J. (1989a). Cultural variations in the response to psychiatric disorders and emotional distress. *Social Science and Medicine, 29*(3), 327–339.

Kirmayer, L. J. (1989b). Psychotherapy and the cultural concept of the person. *Santé, Culture, Health, 6*(3), 241–270.

Kirmayer, L. J. (1991). The place of culture in psychiatric nosology: Taijin kyofusho and DSM-III-R. *Journal of Nervous and Mental Disease, 179*(1), 19–28.

Kirmayer, L. J. (1994). Pacing the void: Social and cultural dimensions of dissociation. In D. Spiegel (Ed.), *Dissociation: Culture, mind and body* (pp. 91–122). Washington, DC: American Psychiatric Press.

Kirmayer, L. J. (1996a). Confusion of the senses: Implications of ethnocultural variations in somatoform and dissociative disorders for PTSD. In A. J. Marsella, M. J. Friedman, E. T. Gerrity, & R. M. Scurfield (Eds.), *Ethnocultural aspects of posttraumatic stress disorders: Issues, research and clinical applications* (pp. 131–164). Washington, DC: American Psychological Association.

Kirmayer, L. J. (1996b). Landscapes of memory: Trauma, narrative and dissociation. In P. Antze & M. Lambek (Eds.), *Tense past: Cultural essays on memory and trauma* (pp. 173–198). London: Routledge.

Kirmayer, L. J., & Robbins, J. M. (1991). Three forms of somatization in primary care: Prevalence, co-occurrence and sociodemographic characteristics. *Journal of Nervous and Mental Disease, 179*(11), 647–655.

Kirmayer, L. J., Robbins, J. M., Dworkind, M., & Yaffe, M. (1993). Somatization and the recognition of depression and anxiety in primary care. *American Journal of Psychiatry, 150*(5), 734–741.

Kirmayer, L. J., & Young, A. (in press). Culture and somatization: Clinical, epidemiological and ethnographic perspectives. *Psychosomatic Medicine.*

Kirmayer, L. J., Young, A., Galbaud du Fort, G., Weinfeld, M., & Lasry, J.-C. (1996). *Pathways and barriers to mental health care: A community survey and ethnographic study* (Working Paper 6). Montreal: Culture & Mental Health Research Unit, Institute of Community & Family Psychiatry, Sir Mortimer B. Davis—Jewish General Hospital.

Kirmayer, L. J., Young, A., & Robbins, J. M. (1994). Symptom attribution in cultural perspective. *Canadian Journal of Psychiatry, 39*(10), 584–595.

Kitanishi, K. (1990). Morita therapy from a transcultural psychiatric view. *Journal of Morita Therapy, 1*(2), 190–194.

Kleinman, A. (1988). *The illness narratives.* New York: Basic Books.

La Via, M., Munno, I., Lydiard, R. B., Workman, E. W., Hubbard, J. R., Michel, Y., & Paulling, E. (1996). The influence of stress intrusion on immunodepression in generalized anxiety disorder patients and controls. *Psychosomatic Medicine, 58,* 138–142.

Lazarus, R. S. (1991). *Emotion and adaptation.* New York: Oxford University Press.

Lewis-Fernandez, R. (1995). *Ataques de nervios in cultural context.* Paper presented at the annual meeting of the Society for Psychological Anthropology, San Juan, Puerto Rico.

Lin, K.-M., Lau, J. K. C., Yamamoto, J., Zheng, Y.-P., Kim, H.-S., Cho, K.-H., & Nakasaki, G. (1992). Hwa-byung: A community study of Korean Americans. *Journal of Nervous and Mental Disease, 180*(6), 386–391.

Lock, M. (1990). On being ethnic: The politics of identity breaking and making in Canada, or, never on Sunday. *Culture, Medicine and Psychiatry, 14*(2), 237–254.

Logue, M. B., Thomas, A. M., Barbee, J. G., Hoehn-Saric, R., Maddock, R. J., Schwab, J., Smith, R. B., Sullivan, M., & Beitman, B. D. (1993). Generalized anxiety disorder patients seek evaluation for cardiological symptoms at the same frequency as patients with panic disorder. *Journal of Psychiatric Research, 27*(1), 55–59.

Low, S. (1994). Embodied metaphors: Nerves as lived experience. In T. Csordas (Ed.), *Embodiment and experience: The existential ground of culture and self* (pp. 139–162). New York: Cambridge University Press.

MacLean, P. D. (1980). Sensory and perceptive factors in emotional functions of the triune brain. In A. O. Rorty (Ed.), *Explaining emotions* (pp. 9–36). Berkeley: University of California Press.

Manson, S., Beals, J., O'Nell, T., Piasecki, J., Bechtold, D., Keane, E., & Jones, M. (1996). Wounded spirits, ailing hearts: PTSD and related disorders among American Indians. In A. J. Marsella, M. J. Friedman, E. T. Gerrity, & R. M. Scurfield (Eds.), *Ethnocultural aspects of posttraumatic stress disorders: Issues, research and clinical applications* (pp. 255–284). Washington, DC: American Psychological Association.

Markus, H. R., & Kitayama, S. (1991). Culture and the self: Implications for cognition, emotion, and motivation. *Psychological Review, 98*(2), 224–253.

McGoldrick, M., Giordano, J., & Pearce, J. K. (Eds.). (1996). *Ethnicity and family therapy* (2nd ed.). New York: Guilford Press.

Miller, J. J., Fletcher, K., & Kabat-Zinn, J. (1995). Three-year follow-up and clinical implications of a mindfulness meditation-based stress reduction intervention in the treatment of anxiety disorders. *General Hospital Psychiatry, 17*, 192–200.

Mumford, D. B. (1989). Somatic sensations and psychological distress among students in Britain and Pakistan. *Social Psychiatry and Psychiatric Epidemiology, 24*, 321–326.

Reynolds, D. K., & Kiefer, C. W. (1977). Cultural adaptability as an attribute of therapies: The case of Morita psychotherapy. *Culture, Medicine and Psychiatry, 1*, 395–412.

Robin, R. W., Chester, B., & Goldman, D. (1996). Cumulative trauma and PTSD in American Indian communities. In A. J. Marsella, M. J. Friedman, E. T. Gerrity, & R. M. Scurfield (Eds.), *Ethnocultural aspects of posttraumatic stress disorders: Issues, research and clinical applications* (pp. 239–254). Washington, DC: American Psychological Association.

Rosaldo, M. Z. (1984). Toward an anthropology of self and feeling. In R. A. Shweder & R. A. LeVine (Eds.), *Culture theory: Essays on mind, self, and emotion* (pp. 137–157). New York: Cambridge University Press.

Rubel, A. J., O'Nell, C. W., & Collado-Ardón, R. (1984). *Susto: A folk illness.* Berkeley: University of California Press.

Salkovskis, P. M. (1989). Somatic problems. In K. Hawton, P. M. Salkovskis, J. Kirk, & D. M. Clark (Eds.), *Cognitive behaviour therapy for psychiatric problems* (pp. 235–276). Oxford: Oxford University Press.

Simon, G. E., & Von Korff, M. (1991). Somatization and psychiatric disorder in the NIMH Epidemiologic Catchment Area study. *American Journal of Psychiatry, 148*(11), 1494–1500.

Thoits, P. A. (1985). Self-labeling processes in mental illness: The role of emotional deviance. *American Journal of Sociology, 91*(2), 221–247.

Vargas, L. A., & Koss-Chioino, J. D. (Eds.). (1992). *Working with culture: Psychotherapeutic interventions with ethnic minority children and adolescents.* San Francisco: Jossey-Bass.

Weiller, E., Bisserbe, J.-C., Boyer, P., Lepine, J.-P., & Lecrubier, Y. (1996). Social phobia in general health care: An unrecognized, undertreated disabling disorder. *British Journal of Psychiatry, 168*, 169–174.

Weissman, M. M., Klerman, G. L., Markowitz, J. S., & Ouellette, R. (1989). Suicidal ideation and suicide attempts in panic disorder and attacks. *New England Journal of Medicine, 321*, 1209–1214.

Weissman, M. M., Markowitz, J. S., Ouellette, R., Greenwald, S., & Kahn, J. P. (1990). Panic disorder and cardiovascular/cerebrovascular problems: Results from a community survey. *American Journal of Psychiatry, 147*(11), 1504–1508.

Wellenkamp, J. (1995). Cultural similarities and differences regarding emotion disclosure: Some examples from Indonesia and the Pacific. In J. W. Pennebaker (Ed.), *Emotion, disclosure, and health* (pp. 293–309). Washington, DC: American Psychological Association.

West, C. (1993). *Race matters.* Boston: Beacon Press.

Wierzbicka, A. (1992). *Semantics, culture, and cognition: Universal human concepts in culture-specific configurations*. New York: Oxford University Press.

Wikan, U. (1990). *Managing turbulent hearts: A Balinese formula for living*. Chicago: University of Chicago Press.

Young, A. (1995). *Harmony of illusions: Inventing posttraumatic stress disorder*. Princeton, NJ: Princeton University Press.

Zajonc, R. B. (1984). On the primacy of affect. *American Psychologist, 39*(2), 117–123.

Zinbarg, R. E., Barlow, D. H., Liebowitz, M., Street, L., Broadhead, E., Katon, W., Roy-Byrne, P., Lepine, J.-P., Teherani, M., Richards, J., Brantley, P. J., & Kraemer, H. (1994). The DSM-IV field trial for mixed anxiety–depressive disorder. *American Journal of Psychiatry, 151*(8), 1153–1162.

Index

94834